INTUITIVE EATING

Respect Your Body and Honor Your Health by Nourishing Yourself Properly

By

Holly Emily Walker

This document is geared towards providing exact and reliable information about the topic and issue covered. The publication is sold with the idea that the publisher is not required to render accounting, officially permitted, or otherwise, qualified services. If advice is necessary, legal or professional, a practiced individual in the profession should be ordered.

From a Declaration of Principles, which was accepted and approved equally by a Committee of the American Bar Association and a Committee of Publishers and Associations.

In no way is it legal to reproduce, duplicate, or transmit any part of this document in either electronic means or printed format. Recording of this publication is strictly prohibited and any storage of this document is not allowed unless with written permission from the publisher. All rights reserved.

The information provided herein is stated to be truthful and consistent, in that any liability, in terms of inattention or otherwise, by any usage or abuse of any policies, processes, or directions contained within is the solitary and utter responsibility of the recipient reader. Under no circumstances will any legal responsibility or blame be held against the publisher for any reparation, damages, or monetary loss due to the information herein, either directly or indirectly.

Respective authors own all copyrights not held by the publisher.

The information herein is offered for informational purposes solely and is universal as so. The presentation of the information is without a contract or any type of guarantee assurance.

The trademarks that are used are without any consent and the publication of the trademark is without permission or backing by the trademark owner. All trademarks and brands within this book are for clarifying purposes only and are owned by the owners themselves, not affiliated with this document.

TABLE OF CONTENTS

INTRODUCTION

In some ways, I was super lucky when I was a teenager. Nobody I knew at school talked about weight or bodies. Maybe it was because I didn't hang with the kids who did. Or, maybe, people just weren't so body focused.

For you, though, it's likely that many of your friends are obsessed with something called the culturally thin ideal. We live in a world that promotes being thin as a lofty goal. Because of this, you're probably hearing a lot of body-bashing comments people saying nasty things about the size or shape of their bodies, because they think they don't match up. Kids of all genders feel the pressure for body perfection.

They talk about how they're sure life would be so much better if only they could buy clothes in a smaller size. Or you may hear them saying that they believe they'd be more popular if they had "Six-packs." Essentially, all teens can be affected by an appearanceoriented world. Regardless of where they fall on the gender spectrum, many teens are victims of these unrealistic demands, they are hating their bodies and fantasizing that they'll be liked or admired more if only their bodies were "Perfect."

It is not surprising that this kind of thinking is so widespread among kids. Adults often think and feel the same way. Your mother may talk about how fat she feels or how she wishes she could just not eat any carbs (as if this were a positive goal!); your father may be upset that he doesn't have the taut muscles he had in college. And even if your parents aren't talking this way, you may hear your doctor say things like, "I'm worried about your weight, you've gained too much this year." That can make you feel bad and inadequate and even scared.

You're also seeing magazine ads using photoshopped pictures of models that look perfect to you, making you feel even more inadequate, and you're bombarded by images of unrealistically thin and flawlessly muscular bodies on TV and in the movies. And then there's social media: a constant reminder that you're not good enough. Social media celebrities and even your friends post pictures of themselves looking as if they have perfect lives. (Of course, people post those pictures only on their best days. And, like everyone, they've probably deleted all the ones on their phones that they think make them look bad and they would never post those!)

Instead of questioning these images or any of the conversations that are going on about this drive for beauty, thinness, and perfection, you may find yourself driven to talk about depressing, anxiety-triggering things like needing to lose weight, debating good versus bad foods, and feeling fat, just as often or even more often than you talk about things that are positive and make you feel happy, like your crushes and your favorite music.

You may believe that you're not good enough just as you are; you may have been tempted to go on diets, so you can get the perfect body. On the other hand, here's the thing: diets are doomed to failure and can have some serious negative side effects, many people who diet go on to bingeing after they fall off the diet. Also, when you hear that someone is on a diet, it's a good bet that there could be a future eating disorder in the making. And what's really scary is that young kids who diet have a big chance of developing an eating disorder by the time they're in their teens.

Sounds like terrible news, right? It does not have to be, because there is another way. Intuitive eating, which you'll be learning about in this workbook, is about being comfortable with who you are, both inside and out, and becoming liberated from the external pressures to conform.

You'll learn what you need to fight the influences social media, TV, movies, your parents, and maybe even your doctor have on you. You'll learn to have a good, healthy relationship with your body and with food in spite of all the messages that make you feel that's just not possible for you.

Intuitive Eating is a philosophy based on the belief that most people are born with all the wisdom they need to know how to eat in a satisfying and balanced way. If you've lost touch with this wisdom and so many of us have Intuitive Eating helps you reconnect with it. It helps you become more body positive and promises you a sense of freedom to truly enjoy all foods and to feel the safety that comes with trusting your wise body.

Over ninety research studies have focused on the benefits of intuitive eating. These studies have shown that intuitive eaters have better coping skills; higher self-esteem; a greater sense of well-being; more optimism, body appreciation, and acceptance; more awareness of signals their body gives them, psychological strength, and unconditional self-regard; and, most important, more pleasure from eating. From a medical standpoint, intuitive eaters are also found to be physically healthier in many ways. So how does this all sound to you? Intriguing, I hope!

The Principles of Intuitive Eating

Intuitive Eating is made up of ten steps or principles:

> ➤ Reject the Diet Mentality. This principle teaches you about what's wrong with dieting and why you're going to want to ditch this miserable process.

> ➤ Honor Your Hunger. Here you'll learn about your personal relationship with hunger. Whether you are usually hungry as a bear, ignore your hunger, or are tuned into normal hunger.

> ➤ Make Peace with Food. Find out if you're living in Food Jail, believing that there are "Good" foods and "Bad" foods. (Hint: there aren't.) And you'll learn to challenge all the rules about eating that have kept you imprisoned.

> ➤ Challenge the Food Police. If you find yourself in Food

Jail, you might need to ask: who is keeping you imprisoned, and how do you free yourself?

➢ Feel Your Fullness. This principle guides you to think about whether you eat and eat until you're uncomfortable and even miserable, and helps you learn why and how to stop eating when you're comfortably full.

➢ Discover the Satisfaction Factor. Just how yummy are your meals? They should be deliciously satisfying. If they're not, this principle sets you on the path to more eating enjoyment.

➢ Cope with Your Emotions Without Using Food. Is food your best friend or your enemy? Maybe it's both. With Intuitive Eating, you'll find ways to separate your emotions from your eating.

➢ Respect Your Body. Is your body your temple, your fortress, or your foe? Here, you'll learn to take loving care of your one and only wonderful body.

➢ Exercise—Feel the Difference. Are you a couch potato or an energizer bunny? Find out how to make movement and activity a happy part of your life.

➢ Honor Your Health with Gentle Nutrition. From nutrition to play food—there's room for it all. It's the key to feeling healthier, happier, and guilt-free!

These principles are usually taught in the order listed above, in this book, though, the order is a bit different because you're a bit different. I decided to teach you about the principles in the order I think will be the most helpful for you, a person whose body and experiences are growing and changing.

CHAPTER ONE
WHAT KIND OF EATER ARE YOU?

P erhaps you are still dieting and don't know it! There are many eating styles, which are actually unconscious forms of dieting. Many of our patients have said they were not on a diet, but upon closer inspection of what and how they eat we found they were still dieting!

Here's a good example. Ted came in because he wanted to lose about fifteen pounds. He said that in his fifty years of living, he had only been on four serious diets. When perusing the book titles in the office (compulsive overeating texts, eating disorder books, and so forth) he stated, "You work with a lot of serious dieting problems ... Well, I'm not one of those." Ted clearly did not see himself as a dieter, merely a careful eater. Yet it turned out that he was an unconscious dieter. Although Ted was not actively dieting, he was undereating to a level where he was nearly passing out in the afternoon.

The reason he had always been unhappy with his weight! In the mornings he would go for an intense hilly bike ride for one hour, then come home and eat a small breakfast. Lunch was usually salad with iced tea (while this sounds healthy, it's too low in carbohydrates). By suppertime, his body would be screaming for food. Ted was not only in a severe calorie deficit, but also carbohydrate-deprived. Evenings turned into a food fest! Ted had thought he had a "Food Volume" problem with a strong sweet tooth. In reality, he had an unconscious diet mentality that biologically triggered his night eating and sweet tooth.

Alicia also was not a conscious dieter. She came in not to lose weight, but because she wanted to increase her energy level. During the initial session, it became clear that she had complicated issues with food. So she was asked if she had been dieting a lot.

She looked astonished. "How did you know that I've been on zillions of diets?" While Alicia claimed to be okay with her current weight, she was still at war with food; she didn't trust herself with food. As it turns out, Alicia had been dieting since she was a child. Although she was not officially dieting, she retained (and expanded) a set of food rules with each diet that nearly paralyzed her ability to eat normally. We see this all the time, the hangover from dieting: Avoiding certain foods at all costs, feeling out of control the moment a "Sinful" food is eaten, feeling guilty when self-imposed food rules are broken, such as "Thou shall not eat past 6:00 p.m."), and so on.

Unconscious dieting usually occurs in the form of meticulous eating habits. There can be a fine line between eating for health and dieting. Notice how even the frozen diet foods such as Lean

Cuisine and Weight Watchers are putting their emphasis on health rather than diet. As long as you are engaged in some form of dieting, you won't be free from food and body worries. Whether you are a conscious or an unconscious dieter, the side effects are similar the diet backlash effect. This is characterized by periods of careful eating, "Blowing It," and paying penance with more dieting or extra-careful eating.

In this chapter, we will explore the various dieting/eating styles to help see where you are now. Later, you will meet the Intuitive Eater and the Intuitive Eating style, the solution to living without diets.

The Eating Personalities

To help you clarify your eating (or dieting) style, we have identified the following key categories of eaters that exhibit characteristic eating patterns: the Careful Eater, the Professional Dieter, and the Unconscious Eater. These eating personalities are exhibited even when you are not officially dieting. It's possible to have more than one eating personality; although we find that there tends to be a dominant trait. Events in your life can also influence or shift your eating personality. For example, one client, a tax attorney, was normally a Careful Eater, but during tax season he became the Chaotic Unconscious Eater.

There's nothing wrong with possessing the eating characteristics described under the three eating personalities. On the other hand, when your eating exists in one of these domains most of the time, it can be a problem.

Read through each eating personality and see which one best reflects your eating style, by understanding where you are now, it will be easier to learn how to become an Intuitive Eater. For example, you may find you have been engaged in a form of dieting, and not even have been aware of it. Or you may discover traits that unknowingly work against you.

The Careful Eater

Careful Eaters are those who tend to be vigilant about what foods they put into their bodies. Ted was an example of a Careful Eater (by day). On the surface, Careful Eaters appear to be "Perfect" eaters. They are highly nutrition-conscious, outwardly, they seem health and fitness-oriented (noble traits admired and reinforced in our society).

Eating Style

There is a range of food behaviors that the Careful Eater exhibits. At one extreme, the Careful Eater may anguish over each morsel of food allowed into the body. Grocery shopping trips are spent scrutinizing food labels. Eating out often means interrogating the waiter what's in the food, how the food is prepared and getting assurances that the food is cooked specifically to the Careful Eater's liking (usually not one speck of oil or other fat used). What's wrong with this? Aren't label reading and assertive restaurant ordering in the health interest of most people? Of course! The difference, however, is the intensity of the vigilance and the ability to let go of an "Eating Indiscretion." Careful Eaters tend to undereat and to monitor the quantity of food eaten.

The Careful Eater can spend most of his or her waking hours planning out the next meal or snack, often worrying about what to eat. While the Careful Eater is not officially on a diet, his or her mind is chastising every "Unhealthy" or fatty food eaten. The Careful Eater can run the fine line between being genuinely interested in health and eating carefully for the sake of body image.

Sometimes the Careful Eater is guided by time or events, for example, some Careful Eaters are meticulous during the weekdays, so that they earn their "Eating Right" to splurge on the weekends or at an upcoming party. On the other hand, weekends occur 104 days of the year, the splurges can backfire with unwanted weight gain. Consequently, it's not unusual for a Careful Eater to contemplate going on a diet.

The Problem

There's nothing wrong with being a Careful Eater and interested in the well-being of your body. The problem occurs, however, when diligent eating (almost bordering on militant) affects a healthy relationship with food and negatively impacts your body. Careful Eaters, upon closer inspection, resemble a subtle dieting style. They may not diet, but they scrutinize every food situation.

The Professional Dieter

Professional Dieters are easier to identify; they are perpetually dieting. They have usually tried the latest commercial diet, diet book, or new weight-loss gimmick. Sometimes dieting takes place in the form of fasting, or "Cutting Back." Professional Dieters know a lot about portions of foods, calories, and "Dieting Tricks," yet the reason they are always on another diet is that the original one never worked. Today, the Professional Dieter is also well-versed in counting carbohydrate grams.

Eating Style

Professional Dieters also have careful eating traits. The difference, however, is that chronic dieters make every eating choice for the sake of losing weight, not necessarily for health. When the dieter is not officially on a diet, he or she is usually thinking about the next diet that can be started. She often wakes up hoping this will be a good day— the new beginning.

While Professional Dieters have a lot of dieting knowledge, it doesn't serve them well. It's not unusual for them to binge or engage in Last Supper eating the moment a forbidden food is eaten. That's because chronic dieters truly believe they will not eat this food again; for tomorrow they diet, tomorrow they start over with a clean slate. Better eat now, it's the last chance. Not surprisingly, the Professional Dieter gets frustrated at the futility of the vicious cycle. Diet, lose weight, gain weight, binge intermittently, and go back to dieting.

The Problem

It's hard to live this way. Yo-yo dieting makes it increasingly difficult to lose weight, let alone eat healthfully. Chronic undereating usually results in overeating or periodic binges.

For some Professional Dieters, the frustration of losing weight becomes so intensified that they may try laxatives, diuretics, and diet pills. And because these "Diet Aids" do not work, they may try extreme methods such as chronic restricting, in the form of anorexia nervosa, or purging (throwing up after a binge), in the form of bulimia.

While anorexia and bulimia are multifactorial and rooted with psychological issues, a growing body of research has demonstrated that chronic dieting is a common stepping-stone into an eating disorder. One study in particular found that by the time dieters reach the age of fifteen years, they are eight times as likely to suffer from an eating disorder as nondieters.

The Unconscious Eater

The Unconscious Eater is often engaged in paired eating which is eating and doing another activity at the same time, such as watching television and eating, or reading and eating. Because of the subtleties and lack of awareness, it can be difficult to identify this eating personality. There are many subtypes of Unconscious Eaters.

The Chaotic Unconscious Eater often lives an overscheduled life, too busy, too many things to do. The chaotic eating style is haphazard; whatever's available will be grabbed vending machine fare, fast food, it'll all do. Nutrition and diet are often important to this person just not at the critical moment of the chaos. Chaotic Eaters are often so busy putting out fires that they have difficulty identifying biological hunger until it's fiercely ravenous. Not surprisingly, the Chaotic Eater goes long periods of time without eating.

The Refuse-Not Unconscious Eater is vulnerable to the mere presence of food, regardless if he or she is hungry or full. Candy jars, food lying around at meetings, food sitting on a kitchen counter will not usually be passed up by the Refuse-Not Eater. Most of the time, however, RefuseNot Eaters are not aware that they are eating, or how much they are eating. For example, the Refuse-Not Eater may pluck up a couple of candies on the way to the restroom without being aware of it. Social outings that revolve around food such as cocktail parties and holiday buffets are especially tough for the Refuse-Not Eater.

The Waste-Not Unconscious Eater values the food dollar. His or her eating drive is often influenced by getting as much as you can for the money. The Waste-Not Eater is especially inclined to clean the plate (and others as well). It's not unusual for a Waste-Not Eater to eat the leftovers from children or spouse.

The Emotional Unconscious Eater uses food to cope with emotions, especially uncomfortable emotions, such as stress, anger, and loneliness. While Emotional Eaters view their eating as the problem, it's often a symptom of a deeper issue. Eating behaviors of the Emotional Eater can range from grabbing a candy bar in stressful times to chronic compulsive binges of vast quantities of food.

The Problem

Unconscious eating in its various forms is a problem if it results in chronic overeating (which can easily occur when you are eating and not quite aware of it).

Keep in mind that somewhere between the first and last bite of food is where the lapse of consciousness takes place. As in, "Oh, it's all gone!" For example, have you ever bought a large box of candy at the movies and begun to eat it only to discover your fingers suddenly scraping the bottom of the empty box? That's a simple form of unconscious eating.

On the other hand, unconscious eating can also exist at an intense level, in a somewhat altered state of eating. In this case, the person is not aware of what is being eaten, why he started eating, or even how the food tastes. It's like zoning out with food.

CHAPTER TWO
WHEN YOUR EATING PERSONALITY WORKS AGAINST YOU

Eventually, the eating styles of the Careful Eater, the Professional Dieter, and the Unconscious Eater become an ineffective way of eating, even when on the surface they appear okay.

The solution for the frustrated eater: Try harder with a new diet! At first the new diet seems exhilarating and hopeful, but eventually the familiar pounds return. Dieting gets more difficult, and even when you resume your baseline eating personality, it may feel more uncomfortable than before.

This is because with each diet the inner food rules get stronger. These food rules often perpetuate feelings of guilt about eating even when you are not officially dieting. Also, the biological effects of dieting make it increasingly difficult to have a normal relationship with food.

The Intuitive Eater personality, however, is the exception. It is the one eating style that doesn't work against you, and can help you end chronic dieting and yo-yo weight fluctuations.

Introducing The Intuitive Eater

Intuitive Eaters march to their inner hunger signals, and eat whatever they choose without experiencing guilt or an ethical dilemma. The Intuitive Eater is an unaffected eater. Yet it is increasingly difficult to be an unaffected eater in today's health-conscious society when you consider the bombardment of nutrition, food, and weight messages from commercials, media, and health professionals.

When we've described the basic eating traits of the Intuitive Eater to our clients, it's amazing how often we'll hear the response, "That's how my wife eats" or "That's how my boyfriend eats." When we ask how that person's weight and relationship to food are, the response is, "No problem!"

Consider Toddlers." They are the natural Intuitive Eaters, virtually free from societal messages about food and body image. Toddlers have an innate wisdom about food if you don't interfere with it. They don't eat based on dieting rules or health, yet study after study shows that if you let a toddler eat spontaneously, he will eat what he needs when given free access to food. (This is probably the toughest thing for a concerned parent to do—to let go and trust that kids have an innate ability to eat!)

A landmark study led by Leann Birch, Ph.D., and published in the New England Journal of Medicine confirmed that preschool-aged children have an innate ability to regulate their eating according to what their bodies need for growth. This holds true even when, meal by meal, the little tykes' eating appears to be a parent's nightmare. Researchers found that at a given meal, calorie intake was highly variable, but it balanced out over time. Yet, many parents assume that their young children cannot adequately regulate their food intake.

Consequently, parents often adopt coercive strategies in an attempt to ensure that the child consumes a nutritionally adequate diet. On the other hand, previous research by Birch and her colleagues indicate that such control strategies are counterproductive.

Furthermore, Birch notes that "Parents' attempts to control their child's eating were reported more often by obese adults than by adults of normal weight." Similarly, Duke University psychologist Philip Costanzo, Ph.D., found that excess weight in school-age children was highly associated with the degree to which parents tried to restrain their children's eating. Even well-meaning parents interfere with intuitive eating, when a parent tries to overrule a child's natural eating cues, the problem gets worse, not better.

A parent who feeds a child whenever a hunger signal is heard, and who stops feeding when the child shows that he's had enough, can play a powerful role in the initial development of Intuitive Eating.

In fact, groundbreaking work by therapist and dietitian Ellyn

Satter has shown that if you get the parents of overweight kids to back off, and let them eat without parental pressure, the kids will eventually eat less. Why? The child begins to hear and understand his own inner signals of hunger and satiety. The child also knows that he or she will have access to food.

According to Satter, "Children deprived of food in an attempt to be thin become preoccupied with food, afraid they won't get enough to eat, and are prone to overeat when they get the chance." We have found this to be true for adult dieters as well. Only for adults, the intuitive eating process has been buried for a long time, often years and years. Instead of having a parent loosen up the pressure, this loosening of pressure has to come from within and against society's myth of dieting and distorted body worship.

Fortunately, we all possess the natural intuitive eating ability; it's just been suppressed, especially by dieting. This book is devoted to showing you how to awaken the Intuitive Eater within.

How Your Intuitive Eater Gets Buried

As toddlers get a little older, mixed messages begin to creep in from the early influences of the Saturday morning food commercial, to the well-meaning parent who coaxes, "Clean your plate." The assault does not stop when you are a child, there are several external forces that influence your eating, which can further bury intuitive eating.

Dieting

You have already seen the damage that chronic dieting plays, including, but not limited to:

- Increased feelings of deprivation

- Increased binge eating

- Decreased metabolic rate

- Increased preoccupation with food

- Increased sense of failure

- Decreased sense of willpower

This only serves to erode your trust with food and urges you to rely on external sources to guide your eating (a food plan, a diet, the time of day, food rules, and so forth). The more you go to external sources to "Judge" if your eating is in check, the, further removed you become from Intuitive Eating. Intuitive Eating relies on your own internal cues and signals.

Eat-Healthfully-or-Die Messages

Messages about eating healthfully are everywhere, from nonprofit health organizations to food companies touting the health benefits of their particular product. The inherent message? What you eat can improve your health? Conversely, take one wrong move (bite) and you're one step closer to the grave. Is this an exaggeration? No. For example, a 1994 press release issued by the

Harvard School of Public Health stated that eating trans fatty acids (found in margarine) may cause 30,000 deaths each year in the United States from heart disease. That kind of message can easily leave you feeling guilty for eating the "Wrong" kind of food and confused about what you should eat.

Magazine and newspapers have also greatly increased their coverage of food and health. One food editor, Joe Crea, of a major metropolitan newspaper, the Orange County Register (California), noted that in a sixyear period (1987-1993) his stories on nutrition increased fivefold. Of nearly eight hundred food stories, two hundred were on health-related issues.

While there is no doubt that what you eat can have an impact on your health, the exponential increase in media coverage has served as a conduit to building food paranoia in the consumer, especially the dieter. Joe Crea agrees, "You open the paper, see a beautiful lead story about cheesecake, and simultaneously another piece on how overeating will make you fat. It puts the reader in conflict."

Are we saying that you should ignore the virtues of healthful eating? Of course, not. However, when you have a dieting mind-set, the barrage of healthy-eating messages can make you feel guiltier about the food you choose to eat. Obesity and Health reported a survey on 2,075 adults in Florida that revealed that 45 percent of adults felt guilty after eating foods they like. (Keep in mind that this survey was conducted to reflect typical American demographics. These "Guilt-by-eating" numbers would most likely be much higher if performed on dieters.)

Women may be especially guilt-ridden. An American Dietetic Association Gallup poll showed that women feel guiltier than men about the food they eat (44 percent versus 28 percent). Could this be because women diet more frequently than men? Or because women are usually the target of health messages and food ads (consider the number of women's magazines). Women are the key decision makers for the health care for the family, and are usually the gatekeepers of food and nutrition issues as well; they serve as a prime target.

We have found that establishing nutrition or healthy eating as an initial priority in the Intuitive Eating process is counterproductive. In the beginning we ignore nutrition, because it interferes with the process of re-learning how to become an Intuitive Eater. Nutrition heresy? No. It's possible to respect and honor nutrition. It just can't be the first priority when you've been dieting all your life. Or look at it this way, if you have focused all your attention on nutrition, has it helped? People can embrace even the most nutritious eating plan (including counting fat grams) as another form of diet.

You can recapture Intuitive Eating, but first you have to get rid of the diet mentality rules that keep the Intuitive Eater buried. In the next chapter, we will briefly introduce you to the core principles of Intuitive Eating. The remainder of the book will show you step by step how to become an Intuitive Eater.

CHAPTER THREE
PRINCIPLES OF INTUITIVE EATING

Only when you vow to discard dieting and replace it with a commitment to Intuitive Eating will you be released from the prison of yo-yo weight fluctuations and food obsessions.

In this chapter, you will be introduced to the core principles of Intuitive Eating, just a snapshot essence of each concept, with a brief case study or two. While in many of these cases, our client's lost weight, the most significant achievement for them was gaining a healthy relationship with food and their bodies. By following the ten principles of Intuitive Eating, you will normalize your relationship with food. How this affects your weight depends on your existing eating style and attitude toward your body.

Later in the book, each principle will be discussed step by step in great detail. You may find it useful to return to this chapter for a quick reference.

Reject The Diet Mentality

Throw out the diet books and magazine articles that offer you the false hope of losing weight quickly, easily, and permanently. Get angry at the lies that have led you to feel as if you were a failure every time a new diet stopped working and you gained back all of the weight. If you allow even one small hope to linger that a new and better diet might be lurking around the corner, it will prevent you from being free to rediscover Intuitive Eating.

James dieted most of his life, starting with the little diets his mother put him on and ending with a liquid protein fast which gave him his most recent short-lived "Success." By the time he came in, James weighed more than he ever had in his life. He knew he was incapable of ever going on another diet, but felt guilty because he thought he "Should." Rejecting the diet mentality was a key milestone for James. He discovered that he was not a failure, but that the system of dieting itself created the setup for failure.

Today, James is a committed ex-dieter who found his way back through Intuitive Eating. He no longer feels that he "Should" be on a diet. He is pleased and amazed that he has lost twenty-five pounds while eating everything he likes. Now, James sadly watches others go from diet to diet while he himself realizes that dieting is the quickest shortcircuit to a healthy relationship with food.

Honor Your Hunger

Keep your body fed biologically with adequate energy and carbohydrates, otherwise, you can trigger a primal drive to overeat. Once you reach the moment of excessive hunger, all intentions of moderate, conscious eating are fleeting and irrelevant. Learning to honor this first biological signal sets the stage for rebuilding trust with yourself and food.

A critical step to becoming an Intuitive Eater for Tim, a busy physician, was learning to honor his hunger. Tim dieted all through medical school while trying to keep up with a frenetic schedule working over eighty hours a week. He felt hungry most of the time, but ignored these signals because he was watching his weight. By midafternoon, his eating was out of control with snack attacks at the vending machine. His weight fluctuated with each dieting attempt and failure. Not surprisingly, he felt low in energy most of the time.

Today, Tim has learned to pay attention to his biological signals of hunger and to honor them by taking the time to feed himself. He knows now that if he doesn't listen to his growling stomach and eat breakfast before he leaves for work, he can't concentrate on what his patients are saying during their morning appointments. Tim has learned to honor his hunger.

As a result of becoming an Intuitive Eater, Tim feels full of energy throughout the day and is back to his college weight (maintaining a fifteenpound weight loss). He has ended the cycles of restriction and overeating that plagued him for twenty years and feels confident that this futile cycle is gone forever.

Make Peace With Food

Call a truce; stop the food fight! Give yourself unconditional permission to eat. If you tell yourself that you can't or shouldn't have a particular food, it can lead to intense feelings of deprivation that build into uncontrollable cravings and, often, bingeing. When you finally "Give in" to your forbidden foods, eating will be experienced with such intensity, it usually results in Last Supper overeating and overwhelming guilt.

Nancy is a waitress whose battleground was a gourmet restaurant offering an array of delicious, rich foods. Before becoming an Intuitive Eater, Nancy would valiantly refrain from all of the tempting foods available at the restaurant. She would leave each night, physically tired and with haunting visions of the foods she shouldn't have. Her restraint was consistent, until making her first appointment. Suddenly, in the week prior to her coming in, all she wanted to do was eat. And eat, she did!

Nancy experienced the Last Supper effect that accompanies intense food deprivation. She had an eating backlash from not allowing herself to touch her favorite foods. Nancy believed that any nutritionist would confirm that she had to give up these foods for good and follow a rigid meal plan. She acknowledged feeling scared and angry about her future food loss and automatically went into a phase of overeating, especially foods that she perceived would be forbidden forever.

Now, that Nancy is an Intuitive Eater, she eats whatever appeals to her at the restaurant and elsewhere. She no longer restricts the foods she likes, nor does she overeat and feel guilty. She discovered that some of the foods that looked wonderful didn't even taste good! Nancy has made peace with food, and loves the freedom that comes with it.

Challenge The Food Police

Scream a loud "No" to thoughts in your head that declare you're "Good" for eating under 1,000 calories or "Bad" because you ate a piece of chocolate cake. The Food Police monitor the unreasonable rules that dieting has created. The police station is housed deep in your psyche and its loudspeaker shouts negative barbs, hopeless phrases, and guilt-provoking indictments. Chasing the Food Police away is a critical step in returning to Intuitive Eating.

As an adolescent, Linda had been a competitive track sprinter and went on to qualify for the Olympic trials. Linda's coach had been a strong influence in her life, and to this day, her coach's voice reverberates, "To be competitive, you must diet to get rid of body fat." She can also hear her mother's voice chiming in about which foods are "Good" and "Bad."

Years of weight fluctuations resulted from obeying the monotonous dieting tapes droning in her head. These inner tapes culminated from her well-meaning coach and numerous diets, only to be reinforced with negative messages that her mother doled out. Linda's Food Police strengthened with each diet, each coaching admonishment, and each motherly chastisement.

Linda's breakthrough came when she discovered how to challenge the Food Police. Linda learned to talk back to the inner critical voices that tried to restrict her food choices. She learned to give herself nurturing messages and make nonjudgmental decisions about her eating.

The voice of the Intuitive Eater was allowed to re-emerge once the Food Police was silenced. Linda is now guilt-free about her eating, and her weight has stabilized at its natural level without dieting.

Feel Your Fullness

Listen for the body signals that tell you you are no longer hungry. Observe the signs that show you're comfortably full. Pause in the middle of eating and ask yourself how the food tastes, and what your current fullness level is.

Jackie was a party girl. She loved to go out to eat with her friends every night after work and felt that weekends were not complete without a party. Jackie loved life and loved to eat. On the other hand, she also didn't know how to stop eating when she began to feel full. (Rather, she often did not recognize feeling full until she was uncomfortably satiated, stuffed.) The morning after each social event she made the same vow: "I never want to eat again. I feel sick and stuffed and bloated, and I hate this roll around my middle."

Learning to feel fullness was a key element in Jackie's journey to Intuitive Eating. She began to pay attention to the transition from an empty stomach to a slightly full stomach. She soon learned to sense the signals of fullness that started to emerge in the midst of her meals.

It was easier for Jackie to honor her body's satiety signals when she truly knew she could eat again if hungry (even within the hour), and eat her favorite foods. (What starving person would stop at comfortable fullness if he thought he was never going to eat again, or have access to a particular food?) Jackie made an interesting observation during one of her out-of-town parties, while feeding alley cats: The starving alley cat will eat until the bowl is licked clean, unlike finicky cats, they know they will be fed again, so they can easily turn up their tails and leave food in their dish. Finicky cats can honor fullness because they know they will eat again.

Jackie also discovered that by honoring satiety signals and pushing her plate away (when she was ready) she was showing more respect for herself. After becoming an Intuitive Eater, Jackie felt that she had it all. She could still go out with her friends whenever she liked, and she could wake up the next morning feeling great!

Discover The Satisfaction Factor

The Japanese have the wisdom to keep pleasure as one of their goals of healthy living. In our fury to be thin and healthy, we often overlook one of the most basic gifts of existence, the pleasure and satisfaction that can be found in the eating experience. When you eat what you really want, in an environment that is inviting, the pleasure you derive will be a powerful force in helping you feel satisfied and content. By providing this experience for yourself, you will find that it takes much less food to decide you've had "Enough."

Denise is a movie production assistant who was surrounded by a variety of "Forbidden" foods each day when she went to the set. Instead of giving herself permission to eat what she really wanted, she would ignore her preference signals.

If she wanted french fries, she would nobly substitute an austere baked potato, unadorned. If cookies beckoned, she'd settle for fruit. Rather than stopping at her substitute food choice, however, she'd continue to seek out food after food, trying to find satisfaction in low-fat foods. Denise couldn't understand why she wasn't losing weight, especially since she was choosing only lean foods.

Once Denise realized that all of these alternate food choices were only fillers, that none of them led her to feel satisfied, she decided to experiment: Eat what she was craving. She was delighted to find that not only did she get true pleasure from the food, but she stopped eating as soon as she finished the portion. Sometimes even leaving some behind! She was satisfied and content not needing to seek out a replacement for her "Phantom Food." Denise discovered the satisfaction factor in eating. She eats far less than ever before, and has lost the weight she struggled with for years. Denise experienced the benefits of our motto, "If you don't love it, don't eat it, and if you love it, savor it."

Cope With Your Emotions Without Using Food

Find ways to comfort, nurture, distract, and resolve your issues without using food. Anxiety, loneliness, boredom, and anger are emotions we all experience throughout life. Each has its own trigger, and each has its own appeasement. Food won't fix any of these feelings. It may comfort for the short term, distract from the pain, or even numb you into a food hangover, but food won't solve the problem. If anything, eating for an emotional hunger will only make you feel worse in the long run. You'll ultimately have to deal with the source of the emotion, as well as the discomfort of overeating.

Marsha was a writer who did most of her work at home. She loved her work, but sometimes found that she would have mini periods of writer's block. To relieve her tension about finding the right word to put on the computer, she would visit the kitchen many times during the day to get a snack. Marsha was using food to help her get her work done.

Lisa was a fourteen-year-old who would come home after school and plop herself down in front of the TV with a bag of potato chips. Lisa was using food to procrastinate doing her homework.

Cynthia's children were grown; she had an illness that depleted her energy, not allowing her to go to work, and her husband didn't pay much attention to her. Cynthia found food to keep her occupied when she was bored and to soothe her lonely soul.

Using food to cope with emotions comes in degrees of intensity.

For some, food is simply a means of distraction from boring activities or a filler for empty times. For others, it can be the only comfort they have to get through a painful life.

Before becoming Intuitive Eaters, Marsha, Lisa, and Cynthia were coping with their problems by using food as a distracter, comforter, and calmer. On the other hand, they soon learned to savor the foods they had chosen, to eat in an inviting environment, and to honor their biological hungers. Increased gratifying eating experiences allowed each to let go of using food as a coping mechanism. They also offered clarity, it was easier to distinguish an eating urge from an emotional urge.

These women discovered that food never tasted as good or was as satisfying when they weren't really hungry, or hadn't figured out what they really wanted to eat, or bolted food down without respecting fullness. Marsha, Lisa, and Cynthia learned to cope without using food and to find appropriate outlets for their emotions. Now they save their eating for the times it gives them true satisfaction, and eat far smaller quantities of food.

Respect Your Body

Accept your genetic blueprint. Just as a person with a shoe size of eight would not expect realistically to squeeze into a size six, it is equally futile and uncomfortable to have a similar expectation about body size. Respect your body so you can feel better about who you are. It's hard to reject the diet mentality if you are unrealistic and overly critical of your body shape.

One of the most important goals that Andrea had while working toward becoming an Intuitive Eater, was to respect her body. She was fifty years old, had given birth to four children, and was a valuable member of the community. Her body had gotten her through childbirth, traveling, working, and exercise. It was a body to respect rather than belittle. Yet, Andrea spent many of her waking hours criticizing her body and remembering the days when she was younger and thinner.

The more she made negative comments to herself, the more despair she felt. She would turn to food when she wasn't hungry to console herself for her misery. She also found herself overeating as a way to punish herself for looking so "Bad."

Once Andrea stopped comparing herself to every other woman she knew and started to respect and honor her body, she began to eat less and to take better care of herself. Andrea became an Intuitive Eater, lost weight, took pride in her achievements, and stopped trying to have the "Perfect" body. Janie, a twenty-five-year-old publicist, also played the Body-check" game. Every time she was at a party, she silently compared herself to other women, only to feel that she was the heaviest woman in attendance. Ironically, Janie had a very fit build, but felt mortified each time and would vow that night to begin a diet the next day. Only when Janie began to focus on respecting her body and its inner cues rather than external forces what other people look like, what other people are doing) did she make a significant breakthrough.

Exercise Feel The Difference

Forget militant exercise. Just get active and feel the difference. Shift your focus to how it feels to move your body, rather than the calorie-burning effect of exercise. If you focus on how you feel from working out, such as energized, it can make the difference between rolling out of bed for a brisk morning walk or hitting the snooze alarm. If when you wake up your only goal is to lose weight, it's usually not a motivating factor in that moment of time.

Miranda had all the accoutrements of a regular exercisera membership in a gym, a stationary bike at home, athletic clothes and shoes. There was just one problem, she was not exercising. Miranda was burned out. She had tried almost as many new exercise programs as she had diets. It was a vicious cycle, begin a diet and simultaneously begin working out, then quit both the diet and the exercise.

That was precisely the problem. Miranda never really felt the pleasure of exercise, of moving her body. Part of the problem was that when she was underfeeding her body (dieting), she had little energy, if any, to exercise and that does not feel good. Consequently, exercising was always a struggle. It was only the initial enthusiasm and momentum of the diet that would carry her through a monotonous workout, but because the dieting was short-lived, so too was the exercise.

When Miranda began feeding her body (by honoring her hunger), she felt better and entertained the idea of beginning a walking program. She discovered that by reframing the purpose of exercise from a weight loss tool to feeling good, she began to actually enjoy walking. For the first time in her life Miranda is consistently exercising and enjoying it. She also knows that she will continue to be consistent because she enjoys the pay-off, which includes feeling better about herself.

Honor Your Health—Gentle Nutrition

Make food choices that honor your health and taste buds while making you feel good. Remember that you don't have to eat a perfect diet to be healthy. You will not suddenly get a nutrient deficiency or gain weight from one snack, one meal, or one day of eating. It's what you eat consistently over time that matters. Progress, not perfection, is what counts.

Louise, like so many of our clients, had dieted all her life. She had been enlightened by the antidieting movement and was ahead of the game with a reject-dieting mentality. On the other hand, Louise had been meticulously counting fat grams like a dieter counting calories, so in essence, she was still dieting. She was using nutrition information militantly to keep herself in check. Her food choices were primarily fat-free foods; they were safe and healthy, she reasoned.

Yet, Louise couldn't understand why she was still bingeing. When Louise realized that she was using nutrition as a dieting weapon, rather than as an ally for health, she began to change the way she chose her foods. Louise honored her taste buds and listened to her body with respect to how food made her feel. When Louise was finally able to relax her eating, to eat with less rigidity, she discovered that it was possible to honor both the pleasure of taste and her health. In addition, by doing this she was more satisfied with eating, her binges ceased, and she was able to attain her natural healthy weight.

A Process With Great Rewards

All of the clients mentioned in the above examples had been dissatisfied with their relationship along food and their bodies. Each had tried either formal or informal dieting and had felt failure and despair. By learning the principles of Intuitive, eating and putting them to work, each found a deepening of the quality of life and resolution about eating. You can too!

CHAPTER FOUR
DEVELOPING AND MAINTAINING A POSITIVE BODY

Combat the effects of pop culture and peer pressure by building self-esteem using these tips to better love yourself. Girls who watch thin, beautiful adult women on TV shows have a more negative body image later on, a study in The British Journal of Psychiatry found.

This research described a cohort of adolescent girls who hadn't been exposed to much television. On the other hannd, after watching it for three or more nights a week, half the teens were more likely to call themselves "Fat" and about a third were more likely to go on a diet than those who didn't watch as much.

It's possible to navigate the rough waters of pop culture and the peer pressure to achieve the "Perfect Body" without developing dangerous body issues. Building self-esteem and taking a stand against negative comments are steps in that direction.

A healthy body image is a difficult thing to define, especially in a culture where it's common for people to casually put themselves down. On the other hand, here's a simple, reasonable definition: "A healthy body image is a body image where you feel happy and confident and accepting of yourself," says Drew Anderson, PhD, an associate professor of psychology at the State University of New York in Albany.

This doesn't mean that you never have a moment of discontent — just that your complaints or concerns about your body, whatever they are, aren't leaving you with body issues that affect your quality of life.

It's important to work toward a healthy body image. Women who have severely negative body images are at greater risk for depression, social isolation, and a host of health problems, such as extreme dieting or eating disorders.

Even though you might not have whatever you think is the perfect body, there is a lot you can do to love the body you are in. Here are some steps you can take toward building self-esteem and appreciating the body you have.

Deconstruct What the Media Is Trying to Present

Learn the facts about what goes into making TV and magazine images of what passes for the perfect body. For example, Anderson says, girls who learn how photographs of stars and models are digitally manipulated before publication often have more positive body images. Also learn about the fashion industry, in particular that models' body types are really dictated by their ability to wear and sell clothes.

Be Realistic About Your Individual Size

The vast majority of people, even those at an ideal weight, cannot measure up to the "Perfect Body" of supermodels or professional athletes. "We have this persistent myth that everybody can be like that if we try hard enough, just buy the right product, work hard enough, etc.," Anderson says. And when you physically can't achieve that goal, "Not only do you dislike yourself, but you also start blaming yourself for not being able to meet that ideal," he adds. You can probably make some important changes, such as working toward a healthy body weight if you are over- or underweight, but you can't turn yourself into a 6-foot-tall, lanky supermodel if you are in fact a curvy, petite, 5'2".

Appreciate The Wonderful Person You Are

"If your whole life is focused on your weight and shape, you're in trouble," Anderson warns. Try shifting your focus to other aspects of your life that you enjoy, whether that's being a good friend, playing a sport you love, or volunteering for a good cause. Make a conscious effort to appreciate the way in which your body, as it is right now, makes it possible for you to enjoy these activities.

Take A Stand When You Hear Fat Jokes

Fat jokes are hurtful while it may be difficult to confront this kind of talk, if someone makes unkind comments about another person's less-than-perfect body, speak up and let them know it's inappropriate. "Be a force of change in your peer group," advises Anderson. For some, this means taking a stand with your family as well. Engaging in fat talk among friends doesn't help body image either. A study of college women published in the journal Psychology of Women Quarterly found that 93 percent of them denigrated their own appearance when they were with their friends.

Anderson adds this advice for parents: Watch your actions. Teens are very sensitive to the divide between what parents say and what they do. Parents who are overly concerned with their own body image or their teen's potential to achieve a perfect body may be adding to body issues, even if they aren't aware of the impact of their words.

When To Get Help

Anderson stresses that periods of dissatisfaction are normal. Additionally, he says, it's entirely possible for anyone a teen or an adult to have a pretty healthy body image, but still want to improve certain aspects, within reason, and that's fine. In addition, you should be aware of certain signals that your body image may be in need of outside help:

When comments are extreme or outrageous It's one thing to say either out loud or to yourself, "Ugh, my hair drives me nuts," but quite another to regularly announce with moody sincerity, "I'm hideous."

When you avoid activities you used to enjoy People can dislike parts of their body, but still have a good time at the beach or a dance. You probably need professional help if you can't go to and enjoy social occasions because of your body issues.

When you engage in extreme diets or workouts Changing your lifestyle to be healthier and improve parts of your body is fine, but going on crash diets, working out excessively, or going to other extremes to achieve your body image ideal is not.

When your expectations are unrealistic Anderson points out that your body type could make it impossible to achieve your ideal or, even if it is possible, it could take months or years, instead of a few weeks of intense work.

When you obsess about certain body parts Body dysmorphic disorder, an extreme form of poor body image, leaves you obsessed about how, in your mind, completely awful certain aspects of your body are, even though other people probably don't even notice the things that concern you.

Remember that whatever body shape you have; you can build a positive body image that allows you to feel great about yourself.

Ways To Shift Your Focus From Losing Weight To Gaining Good Health

If you have tried diet after diet after diet with little success, remember this: "A well-worn path doesn't mean that you are on the right track." If you struggle with weight gain and rarely see positive changes reflected on the bathroom scales, it is important to recognize that the continual diet cycle can do more harm than good—mentally, physically, and spiritually.

The diet cycle typically flows like this:

- We start an extreme diet.

- We feels restricted and deprived.

- The cravings commence and we give into temptation.

- We are consumed with guilt.

- We rinse and repeat this process day in and day out and, for many, year in and year out.

You can absolutely break this dreaded diet cycle and say goodbye to dieting forever by shifting your focus from losing weight to gaining good health.

The following 10 tips will help you to shift your focus.

1. Change the way you set goals

If you struggle with the scales and are always disappointed by your weigh-in results, then take a break from weighing in for a while. Instead of setting goals based on the number of kilos you can lose, set positive change goals.

Positive changes should be celebrated and can include things like eliminating soft drinks permanently, eating more fruits and vegetables daily, enrolling in an exercise class, introducing meditation into your daily routine, walking an extra 10 minutes every day—the list is endless and each positive change that you make is supporting and enhancing your wellness.

2. Stop criticizing yourself

Instead of focussing on all that is wrong with you, focus on all that is right with you. Instead of criticizing your shape and your waistline, start focussing on all of your positive qualities. Find ways to nourish and support your body and acknowledge that every curve, every scar, and every part of you is uniquely you and makes up your amazing story.

Remember that one size does not fit all

We are all wired differently, so what suits one person may not suit the next person, especially when it comes to diet and exercise. Find what suits you personally and focus on making those changes.

4. Listen to your body

Your body is constantly communicating with you. Are you paying attention?

When you really listen to the signs and symptoms your body is giving you, whether it be hunger, pain, or fatigue, you are actually developing an understanding of what it needs and when it needs it. Instead of focussing on losing, focus on listening.

5. Embrace healthy eating as a lifestyle

Lets face it, diets may work in the short term and we may lose a few kilos in the process, but more often than not, when we stop the diet we gain back the weight we have lost and then some. When you accept that healthy eating should be a lifestyle 7 days a week and not a short-term way to achieve weight loss, you will see results. Focus on permanent changes that will last a lifetime.

6. Celebrate your success

As you make changes and start to feel healthier and more energized, really focus on all of the wonderful steps forward you have taken. When you focus on the positive changes you have made and the goals achieved, this is a surefire way to stay motivated. It will fuel you to make even more healthy changes.

7. Shop the perimeter of the supermarket

Instead of heading up and down the supermarket aisles and focussing on low-fat, pre-packaged diet foods as a way to lose weight, change direction. Make the commitment to only shop the perimeter of the supermarket. This is where you will find all the fresh produce—and fresh is always best.

8. Respect your body

Extreme dieting can do more harm than good, so understand that your body must go the distance. Really focus on all that your body does for you and then fuel it accordingly.

9. Remember: Mind + Body+ Spirit

The mind, body, and spirit work as a system of energy, so it is vital to manage all aspects of your wellness. From healthy food and exercise to managing stress levels to factoring in activities daily that uplift your spirit, focus on your system as a whole. It definitely takes a lot more than just eating a salad to achieve good health. Your focus should be on attaining wellness on every level—not just on the scales.

10. Love your body

The more we learn to love our bodies, the more motivated we will be to exercise and eat well. Focus on what you love about your body and not what bugs you.

Here's a tip:

It is not acually our bodies that need to change, but our mindsets and choices. Focus on achieving good health, good energy, wellness, happiness, more joy, more peace, and more love instead of losing more kilos. Remember, your size and weight do not measure your worth as a person, your beauty, your unique qualities, or your contributions to the world. Focus on being the healthiest version of you as a way to move forward.

CHAPTER FIVE
THE SENSUAL EATING
QUALITIES OF FOODS

To discover what foods you really like, and how to increase satisfaction in your eating, explore the sensual qualities of foods. For most people, this means a conscious period of experimentation. Take your taste buds and palate for a sensory joy ride.

Before you eat, consider:

• AROMA

Sometimes the aroma of a food will have more of an effect on your desire for it than does its taste or texture. Appreciate the various aromas that foods can emit. Walk by the bakery and smell the yeasty bread coming out of the oven, or inhale the coffee vapors as the coffee is dripping through the filter. If the aroma of a food is not appealing, you probably won't get your optimal satisfaction from it. If it smells great to you as it is cooking or served to you, however, it will probably increase your satisfaction.

• TASTE

Put a particular food in your mouth to see which of your taste sensations gets stimulated. Roll the food around on your tongue to see if it's predominantly sweet, salty, sour, or bitter. Is that taste pleasant, neutral, or maybe even offensive? Try this experiment at various times during the day to see if certain tastes are more pleasurable at different times. Some people are drawn to the sweet taste at breakfast and want waffles or pancakes. Something spicy, such as eggs with salsa, might be a turn-off early in the morning. Others can't think of something sweet until later in the afternoon.

• TEXTURE

As you roll the food around on your tongue and begin to chew on it, experience the various types of textures that foods can provide. How does crunchy feel to you? Is it abrasive to have to break into a crunchy food, or is it a satisfying experience? What reaction do you have to a food that is smooth or creamy? Does it remind you of baby food, and is that appealing or annoying? Some foods are chewy and require a lot of work by your teeth and tongue. What is that like for you? Sometimes you might just want the flow of a liquid through your mouth and down your throat. Certain food textures might be appealing at different times of the day, or even on different days.

• APPEARANCE

Food artists who design commercial food sets or menus for restaurants know that foods that look appealing are alluring and make a person want to try them. Take a look at the food you're about to eat. Is it attractive to your eye? Is it fresh looking? Is its color interesting to you? Imagine a plate with a poached chicken breast, a boiled potato, and cauliflower—not too thrilling. You'll probably get less satisfaction from that meal than one that's more exciting to look at.

• TEMPERATURE

A steamy bowl of soup might just be the order of the day if it's cold and rainy outside, but chilly frozen yogurt is not usually desirable when you're shivering under an umbrella. Ask yourself what is the most appealing temperature of your foods. Do you like your hot foods boiling hot or temperate? Do you like your cold drinks with lots of ice or very little? Or is room temperature just fine for you for everything?

• VOLUME OR FILLING-CAPACITY

Some foods are light and airy, while others are heavy and filling. The filling capacity of your food choices can make a difference in how much food you need to satisfy you or how you feel after you're finished eating. Some days you might only be satisfied by a plate of pasta which fills your stomach while at other times, a lighter salad is more appealing. Even if something tastes and feels great on your tongue and in your mouth, if it makes your stomach feel queasy or too heavy it will diminish the satisfying experience. Respect Your Individual Taste Buds. Keep in mind that everyone has a different experience with taste and texture sensations. Not all foods will be desirable to you. (If you once got sick on corn, regardless of the cause, corn might never seem appealing again.) Your preferences may be lifelong or may change from time to time. Keep in touch with what is appetizing to you so that you can choose what is most satisfying.

Think About What You Really Feel Like Eating

Once you've gone through this hyperconscious experimentation with the sensory qualities of foods, the next time you feel like a meal or a snack, take a few moments to decide what you really want to eat. If you have trouble deciding what to eat, or need a little clarity, ask yourself:

1   What do I feel like eating?

2   What food aroma might appeal to me?

3   How will the food look to my eye?

4   How will the food taste and feel in my mouth?

5   Do I want something sweet, salty, sour, or even slightly bitter?

6   Do I want something crunchy, smooth, creamy, soft, lumpy, fluid, etc?

7   Do I want something hot, cold, or moderate?

8   Do I want something light, airy, heavy, filling, or in between?

9   How will my stomach feel when I'm finished eating?

If you have a general knowledge of your taste preferences, it will lead you to the right place on the menu or in the supermarket. Checking in with yourself before a meal will give you the specifics of the moment. A further critical key to finding satisfaction in your eating is to take a time-out after you've had a few bites of your food. Is the taste and texture consistent with your desire? Is the food satisfying enough to eat? If you continue to eat a food just because it's there, despite the fact that it's unappealing, you'll only end up feeling unsatisfied when you're finished and find yourself on the prowl for something else that will satisfy you.

Make Your Eating Experience More Enjoyable

Savor Your Food Europeans seem to have cornered the market on slow, sensual eating experiences. Businesses often shut down temporarily to allow for a long lingering lunch, so the meal can be savored and appreciated. Friends tend to gather together to enjoy the conversation and the food. Americans, on the other hand, often engage in desktop dining (fifteen minutes if they're lucky) while going over notes for a meeting. Who do you think has the most satisfying meal experience? Alice is an executive in a company that stresses high productivity. Taking time to sit down for lunch is unheard of, and she's so anxious to get into the office in the morning to begin her calls to the East Coast that she never allows herself to eat breakfast at home before she leaves.

By the time Alice gets home in the evening, the frenetic pace of her day has become a part of her, she ends up gulping down her entire dinner before her husband and daughter get through their salads.

When you race through your meals as Alice does, you don't give yourself the opportunity to experience the sensual aspects of your food. You don't have time to appreciate the attractiveness of the different colors and shapes of the food. You can barely take in their aromas or feel their textures on your tongue and teeth, let alone savor their taste.

To help you savor your food and get more satisfaction from your meals:

1   Make time to appreciate your food. Give yourself a distinct time allowance for a meal. Even fifteen minutes is better than nothing.

2   Sit down at the table or your desk. Standing at the refrigerator or walking around decreases attention and satisfaction.

3   Take several deep breaths before you begin to eat. Deep breathing helps to calm and center you, so you can be focused on eating slowly.

4   Pay attention to eating as slowly as you can. Remember that your taste buds are on your tongue, not in your stomach. Gobbling your food takes away your chance to really taste it.

5   Taste each bite of food that you put in your mouth. Experience ' the different taste and texture sensations the food can provide.

6   Put your fork down now and then throughout the meal. This will help to slow you down.

7   Feel Your Fullness. Take a time-out in the midst of the meal to check your fullness level. Food won't taste as good or be as satisfying after you've reached the last-bite threshold.

Eat When Gently Hungry Rather Than When Overhungry

If you sit down for a meal when you're so hungry that you could eat a cow, you won't be able to tell the difference between a delicious steak and the cow itself! If you're overhungry, your biological need for energy supersedes your ability to eat slowly and taste what's before you. Likewise, if you begin to eat when you aren't really hungry, it can be difficult to decide whether what you're eating is really what you want and whether it's satisfying.

When you're not very hungry, food is not as compelling. If you find this is true for you, this may be a sign that you're not ready to eat just yet. Wait a little while, until your hunger is somewhat more obvious, and you'll find that you'll have an easier time getting in touch with what you really want to eat.

Eat in a Pleasant Environment (When Possible)

Most people find that they get the greatest satisfaction from their meals by eating them in a pleasing setting. Restaurants spend a great deal of time and money creating an environment that is appealing and will draw people back again and again.

The aesthetics of a restaurant can be as important as the taste of the food. At home, the same thing goes. If you set your table in a pleasing manner (a placemat or tablecloth, pretty china, and so forth), your food enjoyment will increase, but eating while standing or driving can diminish satisfaction. If you eat in the car, you are distracted by the traffic and by having to balance food on your lap.

Avoid Tension

Keep heated fights off-limits at the table. One of the surest ways to decrease your satisfaction in eating is to try to eat when you're having an argument with a family member or friend. You'll probably end up eating faster and might even use your chewing as a way to show your anger. You definitely won't have your focus on the food and might eat everything before you without even noticing it—not a satisfying experience!

Provide Variety

Eating a variety of foods is not only nutritionally wise, but it will give you a much broader and more satisfying eating experience. Many of our clients take pride in keeping empty refrigerators and barren cupboards. They believe that if certain foods aren't around, they'll be less tempted to overeat.

The reality is that a lack of appealing food choices creates a sense of deprivation and promotes a creative food-foraging experience that never seems to produce a satisfying result. Give yourself the gift of keeping a variety of foods around, from soups to pastas to cookies or fruits and vegetables. You never know what you might feel like eating. Finding satisfaction in your eating will be a futile attempt if what you want isn't there.

Don't Settle

You are not obligated to finish eating a food just because you took a bite of it. Yet how often have you tasted what appeared to be a mouthwatering dessert, only to discover it was mediocre and yet you kept on eating? One of the biggest assets of being an Intuitive Eater is the ability to toss aside food that isn't to your liking.

This can be easily done when you are truly tasting and experiencing food, combined with the knowledge you can eat whatever you want again.

For the most part, adopt the motto:

"If you don't love it, don't eat it, and if you love it, savor it."

Order something else, find something different in the refrigerator, or eat the parts of the meal that you like and leave the rest.

For example, Barbara spoke of a meal served to her at a banquet that was comprised of salad, chicken, vegetables, and pasta. She took just one taste of the salad and left the rest when she found that the lettuce was soggy under a sea of dressing that she didn't like. The chicken and pasta were delicious, so she ate most of them. The vegetables were so buttery that they overwhelmed her taste buds, so she left them on the plate.

In her old diet days, she would have eaten only the salad and vegetables, thinking that was the "Diet" way to do it, and she would have left her meal unsatisfied, only to go home in search of something else to eat. Melody is another client who is learning to discard what she doesn't find satisfying. One of Melody's favorite foods is a trademark muffin at a local restaurant. Every time she goes to the restaurant, she savors her muffin and feels satisfied. One day, Melody got the inspired notion to bake the trademark muffins from the restaurant's prepared mix and bake she did. When she took a bite of a freshly baked muffin, she was sadly disappointed. It didn't taste anything like what she had eaten in the restaurant. Melody's connection with her Intuitive Eating allowed her to throw out the muffins, with the conviction that she would only eat them when she could get the "Real Thing."

Does it still taste good?

Have you ever eaten a whole bag of cookies or a whole carton of HaaganDazs? If so, you can probably attest to the fact that the first couple of cookies or spoonsful of ice cream tasted much better than those at the bottom of the barrel. Even the taste satisfaction of a large apple dwindles by the time you get down to the core.

In studies of hedonics to food cues (hedonics is the branch of psychology dealing with pleasurable and unpleasurable feelings), researchers find that continued exposure to the same food results in a decrease of desire for that food. We also see that in our clients. Try your own hedonic experiment. Rate the taste pleasure you get from the first few bites of a food from one to ten—one being the least pleasurable and ten being the most. Then stop halfway through eating the food and check your taste buds. Finally, rate the food when you're down to the last bite.

You're likely to find that the numbers diminish along with the food. Routinely, check in with yourself to see if the food tastes as good as it did when you started. If it doesn't, consider stopping, as your satisfaction level is diminishing by the biteful. Wait until you're hungry again. Food will taste better and you'll be more satisfied. And, remember, no one is going to take that food away from your eating repertoire. You can have it for the rest of your life. So why waste your time and your food on a less than satisfying experience!

CHAPTER SIX
IT DOESN'T HAVE TO BE
PERFECT

We've discussed how taking the time to figure out what you really want to eat, and eating in a favorable environment, can lead you to more pleasurable, satisfying eating experiences. On the other hand, what if this isn't always possible? There will be times when you don't have the option of getting exactly what you want. You might be served a meal at a friend's or relative's house that has little to say for it. Many a client has bemoaned meals made by a mother-in-law or an old friend who might boil the vegetables until unrecognizable or cook the chicken until it's the texture of an old shoe. At those times, remember the principle of thinking in gray rather than in black and white.

Intuitive Eating is not a process that seeks perfection, but one that offers guidelines to a co fortable relationship with food. Remember, most of your eating experiences will be more satisfying and pleasurable than you've experienced in years of diets. It's only one meal you will survive. It's how you jump back into taking care of yourself afterward that makes the difference. Sometimes honoring your hunger is the best you can do. And for many of our patients, that alone is significant progress, but if survival eating occupies most of your experiences with food, your satisfaction factor will most likely be low.

Reclaim Your Right To Pleasurable, Satisfying Eating

If dieting has been a significant part of your life for many years, you may need to make a serious effort to reclaim your right to enjoy your food. You may have been so programmed to eat what you were told, especially foods that have little taste pleasure, that you hardly know where to begin to find satisfaction. Knowing what you like to eat, and believing that you have the right to enjoy food, are key factors in a lifetime of weight control without dieting. If it takes you some time to accomplish all of this, be patient. After all, it's taken you many years to lose your ability to truly enjoy eating.

COPE WITH YOUR EMOTIONS

Without using food find ways to comfort, nurture, distract, and resolve your issues without using food. Anxiety, loneliness, boredom, and anger are emotions we all experience throughout life. Each has its own trigger, and each has its own appeasement. Food won't fix any of these feelings. It may comfort for the short term, distract from the pain, or even numb you into a food hangover, but food won't solve the problem. If anything, eating for an emotional hunger will only make you feel worse in the long run. You'll ultimately have to deal with the source of the emotion, as well as the discomfort of overeating.

Eating doesn't occur in a void. Regardless of your weight, food usually has emotional associations. If you have any doubt, catch a glimpse of food commercials. They push our eating buttons—not through our stomachs, but through the emotional connection.

They imply that in sixty seconds or less you can:

- Capture romance with an intimate cup of coffee.

- Bake someone happy.

- Reward yourself with a rich dessert.

Eating can be one of the most emotionally laden experiences that we have in our lives. The emotional rhythm to eating is set from the first day that the infant is offered the breast or the bottle to quell his crying. It's then reinforced each time a cookie is offered to soothe a scraped knee, or ice cream is eaten to celebrate a Little League victory.

Nearly every culture and religion uses food as an important symbolic custom, from the American Thanksgiving feast to the Jewish Passover seder. Each time a significant life experience is celebrated with food, the emotional connection deepens, from the I-got-the-promotion dinner celebration to the: annual birthday cake.

Likewise, each time food is used for a little wound-licking or comfort, the emotional bond strengthens. Food is love, food is comfort, food is reward, food is a reliable friend. In addition, sometimes food becomes your only friend in moments of pain and loneliness. Our patients are embarrassed that food can become so important that food is their best friend. On the other hand, if you consider how emotionally charged food is, it's no surprise that food can evolve into a special salvo.

When a dieter overeats during rough emotional times (whether periodically or chronically), it is usually obvious that food is used as a coping mechanism. For other dieters, it is not so clear. Some of our clients are emotionally unaware they have not yet learned to identify their feelings. It may not be obvious to them that they are using food to cope.

Sometimes, these clients don't know why they are eating. Often the "Why" is an uncomfortable feeling that has not been discovered. Or they may be engaged in a subtle form of emotional eating, such as boredom eating. Nibbling to kill time between classes or appointments is not emotionally charged, but the results can be the same as using food to numb strong feelings—overeating. The eating experience itself, especially overeating, evokes feelings, and those feelings can affect your ability to eat normally. One of the most detrimental feelings that overeating can stir up is guilt and shame.

Studies have shown that although you might have immediate emotional comfort from eating, the negative rush of guilt that bursts forth is powerful enough to completely wipe out the relief. Becoming an Intuitive Eater means learning to be gentle with yourself about how you use food to cope, and letting go of the guilt. As odd as this may sound, eating may have been the only mechanism you had to get through difficult times in your life. It may also have been an inevitable result of years of dieting and feelings of deprivation and despair that arose from dieting. Dieting itself can trigger emotions ultimately lead to using food which to cope with these feelings—chalk up another vicious cycle caused by dieting.

The Continuum Of Emotional Eating

Food can be used to cope with feelings in a myriad of ways. Using food in this way is not a component of biological hunger, but of emotional hunger. Emotional eating is triggered by feelings, such as boredom or anger, not by hunger. These feelings can trigger anything from a benign nibble to an out-of-control binge. It's important to understand that this coping mechanism lies on a continuum of intensity that begins at one end with mild, almost universal sensory eating to the opposite end with numbing, often anesthetizing eating.

The mildest and most common feeling that food can call forth is pleasure. The significance of receiving pleasure from eating is emphasized in Discover the Satisfaction Factor. This concept is not only critical to Intuitive Eating, but is a normal, natural part of living. Don't underestimate the importance of pleasing your palate. by letting yourself enjoy and appreciate eating, you will actually reduce the amount of food you need to feel satisfied when

62

biologically hungry.

For example, allowing yourself little tastes of the special foods available at Thanksgiving will usually offset overeating. Comfort Just the thought of certain foods has the ability to evoke feelings from a comfortable time or place.

For example, do you ever crave chicken soup when you are sick or macaroni and cheese on dreary days because that's what your mom fixed on these occasions? Those are examples of comfort foods. It's normal to have a repertoire of comfort foods. If you want to curl up with a blanket in front of a fireplace and sip hot cocoa with your dinner, that's fine. Eating comfort foods occasionally can be part of a healthy relationship with food, if you do it while staying in touch with your satiety levels and without guilt. If, however, food is the first and only thing that comes to mind to take care of you when you are feeling sad, lonely, or uncomfortable, it can become a destructive coping mechanism.

Distraction If you go a little further on the continuum of emotional eating, food can be used to distract you from feelings you choose not to experience. Using food to cope in this way can become troublesome, as it can be a seductive behavior that blocks your ability to detect your intuitive signals.

It also can inhibit you from discovering the source of the feelings and taking care of your true needs. Whether you're the teenager who sits in front of the TV with a bag of chips to distract you from the feelings of boredom in doing your homework, or you're an executive who goes through a whole bowl of peanuts on your desk to distract you from the anxiety of an arduous meeting, this kind of eating needs to be confronted. There is nothing wrong with occasionally wanting to distract yourself from feelings. Experiencing your feelings twenty-four hours a day can be tedious and overwhelming, but food is not an appropriate distractor for temporary relief.

Sedation

A more serious form of using food to cope is eating for the purpose of numbing or anesthetizing. One client calls this form of eating a "Food Coma." Another suggests that this kind of eating results in a "Food Hangover." In either case, eating to sedate yourself can be as emotionally dangerous as using drugs or alcohol for this purpose. It keeps you from experiencing any feeling for extended periods of time. It becomes impossible to sense your intuitive signals of hunger and satiety, and it deprives you of the satisfying experience that food can bring to your life. Most people who use food in this way talk about feeling out of control, out of touch with life, and generally zoned-out.

They also have trouble recognizing basic sensations of hunger and fullness. Connie is a young woman who had an abusive childhood. She learned to use food at a very early age as a numbing agent. She continues to sedate herself through the anxiety, fear, and sadness of her present life. Connie's weight can escalate five pounds a week when she is regularly going into her

"Food Comas," but even more frightening than her weight gain is the complete detachment from life that she experiences each time. She isolates herself from her friends, calls in sick to work, and feels completely hopeless about life itself. Connie is learning to utilize other coping tools so that she can improve the quality of her life.

When eating to numb and sedate is occasional and short term, it tends to have little detrimental effect. On the other hand, this kind of eating can escalate into an addictive behavior before you even notice it.

Punishment Sometimes, eating for the purpose of sedation becomes so frequent and intense that self-blame ensues and ultimately triggers punishing behaviors. Clients find themselves eating large quantities of food in an angry, forceful manner that allows them to feel beaten up. This is the most severe form of emotional eating and can lead to loss of self-esteem and to self-hatred. Clients who use food to punish themselves report no pleasure in their eating and actually begin to hate food.

Fortunately, this type of eating behavior disappears when the Nurturer voice can be beckoned to give understanding and compassion. If there's no crime committed, no punishment need be tendered.

Emotional Triggers

We've looked at general emotional reasons for eating; now let's examine the specific feelings involved. A craving for certain foods, or simply a desire to eat can be triggered by a variety of feelings and situations.

Some people use food to cope when they have no idea that's what they're doing. They think that they're overeating "Just because it tastes good." If you find that you're doing quite a bit of eating when you're not biologically hungry, then there's a good chance that you are using food to cope. You may not have deep-seated emotional reasons for eating, but just getting through life's hassles with some of its irksome tasks and boredom might trigger you to seek food to make it all easier.

Boredom and Procrastination

One of the most common reasons people eat when they're not hungry is boredom. In fact, studies have shown that regardless of a person's weight, boredom is one of the most common triggers of emotional eating.

One particular study divided college students into two groups. One group had the monotonous task of writing the same letters over and over again for nearly half an hour. The other group was engaged in a stimulating writing project. Students in each group were given a bowl of crackers to nibble on. Guess which group ate more? Regardless of weight, the "Bored" group ate the most crackers.

In boredom eating, food is used as a way to fill time as well as a way to put off doing mundane work. For some people, the thought of the food and the actual experience of going for it and eating it breaks the tedium. Here are some situations that produce boredom eating.

- Lying around the house on a Sunday afternoon when you've made no plans for the day.

- Having to get through an afternoon of studying, paperwork, or a writing project.

- Watching a boring night of television with nothing else to do, but take food breaks.

- Killing time: waiting for a meeting to get started, waiting for a phone call, and so forth. We also see this type of eating in our overworked clients they feel they must always be doing something, being productive. The moment a tiny hole opens up in their schedule, they feel the need to fill it often with food. (It's acceptable to eat, but not to rest!)

Intuitive Bribery Eating And Reward

Have you ever promised yourself that you could have a treat once you finished writing a term paper or a contract, or cleaning the house? If so, you have experienced reward eating. It's not unusual to use food as a motivation for accomplishing undesired tasks.

For example:

- Children are often bribed with treats such as candy or ice cream if they behave—at the mall, for a baby-sitter, and so on.

- People often reward themselves for working hard: at work, at home, or at school with an extra bagel or a muffin, for example. Using food as a reward can be self-perpetuating, as there will always be ongoing tasks and challenges which can be made more tolerable if they're mitigated by food gifts.

Excitement food and the eating experience itself can serve as a way to add excitement when life begins to feel dull. At a subtle level, planning a special meal or making a reservation at a favorite restaurant can create a sense of excitement. The notion of going on a diet can trigger feelings of hope.

This is one of the reasons why dieting is so alluring. Our clients talk of how even contemplating a new diet gives them a rush of adrenaline—just imagining a new body and a new life. When the diet fails, the excitement is replaced with despair. At this point, the experience of going to the store to buy large quantities of forbidden foods can be one way to recreate the excitement. And then the cycle continues diet/overeating, diet/overeating. This is exciting, but at what cost?

Soothing It's not hard to understand the soothing power that food can provide. It can be more appealing to go to the kitchen for cookies and milk than to sit on the couch and experience uncomfortable feelings. This is daily true if those cookies and milk remind you of a time that was pleasant and life felt less complicated. Habitually eating to soothe what ails you can evolve into a problem with food. Food can have other symbolic associations with comfort. Ellen is a sixteen-year-old who has battled with her father since she was a small child. She describes him as mean and nasty with a bitter personality. It was not surprising to hear Ellen talk about her obsession with eating large amounts of candy every day as a way to bring "Sweetness" into her life. To her, the sweets countered the bitterness of her daily experiences with her father.

Love Food can become connected to the feeling of being loved. There is certainly a romantic link with food—chocolate on Valentine's Day is a classic example. When dating, there's an unspoken ground rule that your relationship is elevated to a more intimate level when you have experienced a home-cooked meal for two. Clients frequently tell of how their parents' only way to show love was through food. These parents may not have been able to show physical attention or speak to them in loving ways, but food was always plentiful.

Frustration, Anger, and Rage

If you find yourself going through a bag of hard and crunchy pretzels when you're not hungry, it's a good bet that you may be feeling frustrated or angry. The physical act of biting and crunching can serve as a way to release these feelings for some people. One client, Nancy, a lawyer, discovered that she had a habit of subduing her anger at some of her clients by grabbing some hard food, whether it was carrots or crackers, and munching away.

Stress many of our clients say they head for the nearest candy bar under stressful times. Yet, in most individuals, biological mechanisms associated with stress turn off the desire to eat.

The rush of adrenaline during stressful times sets in motion a cascade of biological events to provide immediate energy. As a result, blood sugar is elevated and digestion is slowed. These two elements alone tend to suppress hunger and heighten the sense of satiety when eating.

The biological reactions are a form of self-preservation to ready our bodies for "Fight or flight." While this was quite useful for survival, fighting off a man-eating tiger or fleeing from danger required immediate energy—a growing body of research suggests that in our modern day this mechanism may actually contribute to obesity. It may be stressful to fight off rush-hour traffic or to flee from a deadline, but you don't need the extra blood sugar that the stress reaction provides. Where does it go? If you don't use it (in the way of physical activity), excess blood sugar gets converted to fat. This biological problem is only compounded if you cope with stress by eating. Studies have also shown that people who have been dieting are especially vulnerable to overeating during stressful times. Stress becomes one more reason to "Blow" the diet. Dieting itself can also be a source of stress.

Anxiety Worries of any magnitude, from an upcoming final to

waiting to hear if you got the job, can trigger an urgent need to eat to relieve anxiety. Sometimes generalized anxiety can be described as that uncomfortable feeling you are unable to put a finger on; our clients say it feels like butterflies in your stomach. With the focus on the stomach so goes the food.

Mild Depression

It's not uncommon for many people to turn to food when they are mildly depressed. In mild depression weight gain is often seen, especially in dieters. In one study, 62 percent of the dieters and 52 percent of nondieters stated they ate more when feeling depressed.

CHAPTER SEVEN
COPING WITH EMOTIONAL EATING

Whether your response to emotional hunger is mild emotional eating or out-of-control binge, there are four key steps to making food less important in your life.

Ask yourself:

1   Am I biologically hungry? If the answer is yes, your next step is to honor your hunger and eat! If you are not hungry, answer the following questions.

2   What am I feeling? When you find yourself reaching for food when there is no biological hunger, take a time-out to find out what you are feeling. This is not such an easy question to answer, especially if you are not in touch with your feelings. Try the following:

*   Write out your feelings.

*   Call a friend and talk about your feelings.

*   Talk about your feelings into a tape recorder.

*   Just sit with your feelings and experience them if you

can.

- Talk to a counselor or a psychotherapist.

3   What do I need? Many people eat to fulfill some unmet need, which is related to the emotional or physical feeling being experienced. If you are a chronic dieter you can be particularly vulnerable. Eating to assuage an unmet need can be used as an excuse to eat. Here is a simple example: Molly is a freelance writer who was working into the wee hours to meet her deadline. Around 3:00 in the morning she found herself walking downstairs into the kitchen. She realized that she was not hungry, yet she was about to devour a bowl of ice cream. When Molly asked herself what she was feeling, she discovered frustration, exhaustion, and a sense of being brain-dead. She realized that she was trying to feed both her fatigue and her frustration, but what she really needed was rest—no amount of food would replace sleep. She decided to call it a night and go to bed. On the other hand, before Molly made that decision, she told herself she could have the ice cream tomorrow if she still wanted it. She also realized the ice cream would taste better if she experienced it fully awake rather than half asleep. The next day Molly finished her story and had no desire for the ice cream—she had removed the need.

4 Would you please . . . ? It's not unusual to find—when you ask the question "What do I need?"—that the answer can be obtained simply by speaking up and asking for help. Laurel Mellin, innovator of the successful Shapedown weight management program for families, has found that overweight kids often have trouble speaking up for their needs. We find this to be true also for many of our clients. The "Would you please" i step originated from Laurel Mellin's work, and we find it extremely helpful for our clients. Danielle, a full-time stay-at-home mom, learned that she was using food as a momentary time-out. Eating was her only retreat between baby cries. Danielle discovered that what she needed was not food, but time just for herself. To obtain this she used the "Would you please" step. She asked her husband to give her thirty minutes of uninterrupted quiet time after he came home from work. Having gained this, food was no longer so important.

MEETING YOUR NEEDS WITHOUT FOOD

There are various ways in which we learn to handle the unending emotions that life can trigger. Some people learn early on that it's okay to express their feelings or to ask for a hug. Others aren't lucky enough to be taught how to take care of themselves in productive, nurturing ways. The first task in learning how to cope without using food is to acknowledge that you are entitled to

74

having your needs met.

On the other hand, basic needs are often discounted, including:

- Getting rest

- Getting sensual pleasure

- Expressing feelings

- Being heard, understood, and accepted

- Being intellectually and creatively stimulated Receiving comfort and warmth

Seek Nurture

Feeling nurtured can allow you to feel comfort and warmth so that food loses its number-one position in this role. There are many routes and avenues available for nurturing yourself and receiving nurturing from others:

- Rest and relax.

- Take a sauna or a Jacuzzi.

- Listen to soothing music.

- Take time to breathe deeply.

- Learn to meditate.

- Play cards with friends.

- Take a bubble bath in candlelight.

- Take a yoga class.

- Get a massage.

- Play with your dog or cat.

- Develop a network of friends.

- Ask friends for hugs.

- Buy yourself little presents.

- Put fresh flowers in your house.

- Spend time gardening.

- Get a manicure, pedicure, facial, haircut, etc.

- Get a teddy bear and hug it.

Deal with Your Feelings

If you receive a steady flow of comfort and nurturing you'll be better prepared to face the feelings that have been so frightening. Acknowledge what is troubling you—allow your feelings to come up. This will reduce your need to push them down with food.

Here are some suggestions of how to deal with your feelings:

- Write your feelings in a journal.

- Call a friend (or several).

- Talk about your feelings into a tape recorder.

- Release anger through pounding a pillow or a punching bag.

- Confront the person who is triggering your feelings.

- Let yourself cry.

- Breathe deeply.

- Sit with your feelings and discover how the intensity will diminish with time.

- If you have trouble identifying your feelings or coping with them, it may be helpful to talk with a therapist, especially if it is a persistent issue.

Find a Different Distractor

Many people use food as their primary distraction from their feelings. It's okay to get away from your feelings from time to time, but you don't have to use food as an excuse. Many teenagers tell us that they come home from school every afternoon and plop down in front of the TV with a bag of chips and a soda.

When asked why they do this, they say that they're avoiding the boring feelings of having to do their homework. When it's suggested that they first have a snack to take care of their biological hunger and then watch some TV to distract themselves for a while before settling down to homework, they exclaim that their parents would never let them. As long as they're eating, they can legitimately put off doing homework, but having other distractors is not allowed! This is also true for many workaholic clients. It's socially acceptable to take a time-out to eat (a coffee break), but to just sit at the desk, even while entitled to a break, is not allowed. They fear that it will appear as if they are doing nothing. Others use food to distract themselves from loneliness, fear, and anxiety. Since it would be overwhelming to try to feel your feelings twenty-four hours a day, give yourself permission to take a break from them for a while.

Take the assertive stance of distracting yourself in an emotionally healthy way. Try the following:

- Read an absorbing book.

- Rent a movie.

- Talk on the telephone.

- Go to the movies.

- Take a drive.

- Clean out your closet.

- Put on some music and dance.

- Peruse a magazine.

- Take a stroll around the block.

- Work in the garden.

- Listen to a novel on tape.

- Do a crossword puzzle.

- Work on a jigsaw puzzle.

- Play with the computer.

- Take a nap.

How Emotional Overeating Has Hurt And Helped?

As you begin to examine your use of food as a coping mechanism, it's helpful to take a look at how food has actually helped you. The notion that overeating can have benefits may sound crazy to you, especially if you're feeling distressed by this behavior and by your weight, but if there were no up side to overeating, you probably wouldn't continue it. Take a piece of paper and divide it in half. On one half, make a list of "How using food serves me"—cite all the benefits you receive from overeating. Title the other side, "How using food does me a disservice," and examine the ways in which food has become harmful or destructive to you.

A list might look like the following:

- It tastes good.

- It makes me overweight.

- It's reliable—it's always there.

- My clothes don't fit.

- It keeps me from feeling bored.

- I'm uncomfortable walking and exercising.

- It soothes me.

- My cholesterol is high.

- It numbs my bad feelings.

- I'm numbed to the joys of life.

As you look over your list, you might be surprised to learn that the use of food is not just a negative experience for you. In fact, it may give you some valuable perks. On the other hand, if you're feeling bad and guilty about using food to cope it will be hard for you to recognize that its benefits may equalize its burdens. By recognizing that there are indeed some benefits to using food, you'll begin to own your eating experience rather than feeling out of control.

When For Is No Longer Important

Many clients have talked about having strange, uncomfortable feelings when they're no longer using food to cope with their emotions. At the same time, they're feeling happy and secure in their new Intuitive Eating style and may be losing the weight that has always been a struggle for them.

There are a couple of reasons for the conflicting feelings:

- You no longer have the "Benefits" of using food. While coping with food can be destructive, one client noted that on tough days she knew she could always go home to her chocolate. Now, instead, she's "Stuck" with experiencing her feelings. You might even need to go through a grieving period for the loss of food as comforter and companion.

- You may also notice that you're experiencing your feelings in a deeper, stronger way. Since you're no longer covering them up with food, they may have a profound effect on you. This is a point at which some people decide that it would be helpful to get counseling as a way to process these long-buried feelings.

Sandy is a client who experienced the loss of using food as a coping mechanism. By acknowledging what food used to do for her as well as against her, Sandy was able to understand that her uncomfortable feelings were normal and appropriate. Sandy had either dieted or used food to cope all of her life. She talked about feeling very frustrated when she would stop eating after finding the threshold bite and truly not wanting _ any more food. She knew that she'd had enough, didn't want to feel uncomfortable by eating more, yet felt unhappy that she wouldn't be able to continue to have the taste sensations that the food provided. She also talked about feeling angry that she no longer had food to turn to when she was feeling bad. Eating isn't as exciting as it used to be when

Sandy would restrict and then overeat. Soon, however, after mourning the loss of being able to use food, she was able to leave these feelings behind and feel mainly the exhilaration of being an Intuitive Eater who copes without using food.

A STRANGE GIFT

You may go for a long time without using food to cope, when all of a sudden emotional eating catches you by surprise. If this occurs, it's not a sign of failure or that you've lost ground; instead, it's a strange gift.

Overeating is simply a sign that stresses in your life at that moment surpass the coping mechanisms that you have developed. Some of these stresses are divorce, a job change, a move to a new city, the death of someone close, marriage, or the birth of a child. These may be new or unexpected experiences for you.

As a result, you haven't had the opportunity to develop coping skills to deal with them. So, you revert to eating as the familiar way to take care of yourself. Overeating can also recur when your lifestyle becomes unbalanced with too many responsibilities and obligations, with too little time for Z'pleasure and relaxation. Consequently, food is used to indulge, escape, and relax (albeit briefly). When you find this happening, it may be a signal for you to reevaluate your life and find ways to put more balance into I it. If you don't make these necessary changes, food remains important by filling an unmet need. r In both of these situations we've described, overeating becomes a red ' flag that lets you know that something isn't right in your life.

Once you truly appreciate this, eating will not feel out of control, rather it's an early warning system. Recognize how lucky you are to have this mechanism to alert you that something is out of kilter in your life! (At first, our clients think this notion is a bit absurd, until they realize the truth behind it in their own lives.) Those people who have never had an emotional eating problem often have no recognizable warning of excess stress in their lives. If you can see that your eating problem can have benefits as well as bad effects, you won't slip into a pattern of self-defeating behaviors that become destructive and difficult to reverse.

Using Food Constructively

Once you learn new ways of coping with your emotions, think about how food can continue to nurture you in a constructive way. You have a right to feel good and that means not just not feeling stuffed, but also feeling satisfied with your food choices, being healthy now, and reducing future health risks. Your relationship with food will become more positive as you begin to let go of food as a coping mechanism and bring it into your life as a nonthreatening, pleasurable experience. We discuss how you can eat healthfully without falling back into the diet mentality, but first you need to learn how to respect your body and appreciate how it feels when you exercise.

Respect Your Body Accept Your Genetic Blueprint

Just as a person with a shoe size of eight would not expect realistically to squeeze into a size six, it is equally futile (and uncomfortable) to have a similar expectation about body size. Respect your body so you can feel better about who you are. It's hard to reject the diet mentality if you are unrealistic and overly critical of your body shape.

Body vigilance begets body worry, which begets food worry, which fuels the cycle of dieting. So what do you do, just forget it?

Crawl into a dark cave, hide from the world and eat everything in sight? No, but as long as you are at war with your body it will be difficult to be at peace with yourself and food. With every disparaging glance in the mirror, the Food Police gain power, and with that comes vows of just one more diet. Has all the self-loathing because of your body helped? Has dwelling on your imperfect body parts helped you to become leaner, or merely made you feel worse? Does chewing yourself out every time you step on the scale make your weight any less? We have yet to find one client who says that focusing on his or her body in such negative ways is helpful. Studies have shown that the more you focus on your body, the worse you feel about yourself.

Yet the body torture game goes on—Mirror, mirror on the wall, who's the slimmest of them all? It's hard to escape the body torture game when the whole country is playing it. In the name of fitness, a lean and hard shape has become the body icon since the nineties. Self-proclaimed fitness gurus insist that you can "Sculpt" your body as if it were a lump of clay, that you can

Respect Your Body

change your genetic shape with an aerobic huff and puff. We are ardent advocates of being fit and recognize the health benefits of exercise, but we feel we must point out that unrealistic expectations are being painted. It is widely accepted in the research community that you cannot spotreduce (lose fat in just one specified place).

So how could it be that you can sculpt your body by working on certain body parts? Yes, you can build specific muscles through strength and resistance training. And yes, you can lose overall body fat through aerobic exercise, but you cannot personally select where that fat will be lost. It's possible to build muscle underneath fat layers, but this is not the concept of body sculpting that most overweight people have in mind. Most clients we speak with take body-sculpting classes in hopes of chiseling off the fat. The fashion world has shaped the ideal look for women into various versions of thin—from the sixties Twiggy figure to the modern waif look embodied by supermodel Kate Moss. Even the full-bodied fashion look turns out to be too thin by medical standards.

When clothing giant Guess hired model Anna Nicole Smith, she made headlines in the fashion and news media because she was "Big." She weighed 150-155 pounds (gasp), yet was 5'11", which is in the lower range of ideal according to 1990 U.S. height and weight charts! If a normal weight is considered "Big," what does that say about the average woman? This hardly fosters realistic body-shape expectations. If the ideal body type for women is sandwiched between the Spandex fitness look and fashionable waifness, most bodies don't stand a chance. No wonder body dissatisfaction has become the norm in this country. Repeatedly we seem to be sold the message, If they can do it, you can do it; just try harder (after all, even if you are lean, you could still be leaner). With such standards, it's no wonder that women—-and increasingly men, too—are at war with their bodies. Whether you are male or female, fat is the enemy.

There is no doubt that there are unrealistic pressures to be thin, with contributions from the media, advertisers, fashion industry, beauty industry, and on and on. And there are a myriad of cultural factors that lead to unrealistic body expectations. We could groan and point fingers at the causes leading to increased body dissatisfaction. On the other hand, we want to get past the cause and effect analysis, and instead focus our energy on how to get past body vigilance.

Make Exercise a Nonnegotiable Priority

Ask yourself, "When can I consistently make the time to work out?" Make an appointment with yourself to work out, and honor it as you would any other meeting or appointment. If you travel a lot:

- Pack your walking shoes. (It's an interesting way to get to know a new city.)

- Pack a jump rope. (It's a lightweight piece of equipment that delivers a cardio-wallop in a short amount of time.)

- Choose hotels that have workout facilities. (They are increasing in number.)

- Take advantage of airport layovers and walk around the airport. (It usually feels good after hours of sitting.)

Be Comfortable

Workout attire need not be fashion show material, but it is

important to wear clothes that breathe and allow you to move. This also means dressing for the weather. Heavy sweats can make you uncomfortably hot when you wear them to disguise your body. An oversize lightweight T-shirt and leggings will usually do for women. Or bike shorts with an oversize shirt works well for both men and women. Don't forget about comfortable shoes as well. Not only will they feel good; they are an investment in injury prevention.

Include Strength Training

Strength training helps rebuild muscle wear and tear from dieting. This is also important because our lean muscle mass declines as we get older. Americans lose an average of about 6.6 pounds of lean muscle mass for each decade of life. Therefore, someone who has been dieting for years is losing her muscle tissue from both aging and dieting. Remember, muscle is metabolically active tissue that helps keep your metabolism revved up.

In fact, Bill Evans and Irwin Rosenberg, Tufts University researchers and authors of Biomarkers, estimate that our metabolic rate decreases 2 percent each year from the age of twenty, and they attribute this downward shift of metabolism to decreasing muscle mass. Ordinary activity, and even vigorous activity such as running, does not leave you immune to muscle-wasting due to age.

A ten-year study following master runners (minimum age of forty) showed that while they maintained their fitness from running, they lost an average of 4.4 pounds of muscle from their untrained areas. Their muscles stayed the same size in their legs, but decreased in their arms. There was an exception, however, for three runners who did upper body weights. They were able to maintain their fat-free weight in their upper body. Therefore, you don't have to lose your muscle mass.

The American College of Sports Medicine (ACSM) recommends that strength training be an integral part of a fitness program for all healthy adults. Specifically, they recommend:

- Strength training at least twice a week

- Doing one set of eight to twelve repetitions of eight to ten exercises for conditioning of each of the major muscle groups

BEYOND PHYSICAL FITNESS

Is there anything wrong with wanting to work out more, to burn body fat? No. Just be careful that you do not fall into the dieting-weight loss trap, where you become a slave to working out and counting calories burned. We have found that increasing exercise can be a good way to channel anxiety while becoming an Intuitive Eater. Intuitive eating can feel foreign and slow in the beginning, especially when the world around you is dieting.

Exercise allows you to feel that you are actively doing something about your body. You feel benefits. It's one thing to invest several hours in exercise if you are training for a marathon or because you are an athlete. It's a problem, however, when exercise consumes you, and begins to interfere with your everyday living.

Exercising more isn't necessarily better. How do you know if you are reaching the outer limits of exercise?

Signs of exercise abuse include:

- Inability to stop, even when you are sick or injured

- Feeling guilty if you miss a single day

- Inability to sleep at night—a sign of overtraining

- Paying exercise penance for eating too much, such as running an extra three miles because you ate a piece of pie

- Being afraid that you will suddenly get fat if you stop for a single day

RR—REMEMBER REST

The hardest lesson that I learned from a competitive marathoner was that rest was every bit as important as training. It's also hard for our clients to recognize this tenet of training. Similarly, if for some reason you are unable to work out on a particular day, it does not mean that you will be suddenly out of shape or gain weight. Some clients fear that once they stop exercising they will not continue.

That's the all-or-nothing thinking commonly seen in dieters. There's an easy way to prove to yourself that no exercise today does not mean no exercise forever. Simply resume exercise when you are able. The more you reinitiate an exercise program after a break from it, the more confidence you will have in your ability to continue exercising, even if it's been a few days. After a while it stops being a big issue or worry. Besides, this time it's different. You are not dieting, therefore, it will be much easier to resume training. Remember, a few days or weeks of no exercise will not make or break your health or weight.

After the big 1994 Los Angeles earthquake, Diane, a client, had to stop exercising, but for the first time, Diane knew that although three weeks had passed, it wasn't a big deal. She knew she'd be lacing up her walking shoes again in the near future. Diane missed the stress relief; she missed the freedom from the kids, but she also knew that she had a house to rebuild. After the earth settled, she got back to her routine walking. Her missed exercise did not become a crisis, and neither did her weight. Sometimes, taking care of yourself means choosing not to exercise. For example, if you only got four hours of sleep and exercising means rising at five in the morning, it's probably best to take that day off. Remember, rest is important. Likewise, if you feel a cold coming on, or you're feeling worn-out, take a day off. Listen to your body. Rest will also help keep exercise feeling fresh and fun.

The Ultimate Path Toward Healing From Eating Disorders

Eating disorders are not just a fad or a phase. They are serious, potentially life-threatening conditions that affect a person's emotional and physical health. National Eating Disorders Association

A.s you have explored this book, you may have noticed a number of references to eating disorders, especially comments about how dieting has been found to be one of the most provocative and powerful catalysts in the development of an eating disorder. We have yet to meet a patient who declares "I want to have bulimia, anorexia, or a binge-eating disorder." It usually starts off with: "I just want to lose a few pounds," which evolves into dieting, to disordered eating, and, finally, to full-syndrome eating disorders. In fact, 35 percent of so-called normal dieters progress to pathological dieting. Of those, 20 to 25 percent will progress to partial or full-blown eating disorders. In the United States alone, it is estimated that there are five to ten million girls and women struggling with some type of eating disorder.

In addition, there are one million boys and men with an eating disorder. These are conservative estimates from the National Eating Disorders Association, but let's not focus on statistics in this chapter. Instead, let's get into the real lives and painful experiences of some of our patients who have plunged into the world of dieting, have then catapulted into a fullfledged, diagnosable eating disorder, and have ultimately come to work with us in their paths to recovery.

The Ultimate Path Toward Healing from Eating Disorders 215 phy of Intuitive Eating cannot be fully embraced in the beginning of treatment for a serious eating disorder. Most patients who are in the throes of anorexia nervosa, bulimia nervosa, or compulsive overeating have lost touch with their innate signals of hunger and fullness and taste preference. The physical starvation is often so grave in those who are suffering from anorexia nervosa that an attempt to listen to signals of hunger or fullness can only lead to confusion and maintenance of the underfed state. If even the smallest amount of food is ingested, the slowed stomach emptying that occurs in anorexia pushes away signs of hunger and creates a false sense of fullness.

In the early treatment of anorexia, we attempt to refeed patients in a very slow, deliberate fashion, so as not to overstress the body physically or overstress the emotions and create excessive fear. In the treatment of bingeing disorders, including bulimia, patients have become so accustomed to eating quantities of food that are larger than one's normal needs that their interpretation of fullness is highly skewed. They so often have ignored hunger by eating for many other reasons, such as boredom, loneliness, anger, etc., that asking them to listen to hunger signals feels alien and frustrating. We begin, instead, with putting on our nutritionist caps and teaching them about normal body functioning, including the concept of blood sugar fluctuations and the body's reaction to meals that are unbalanced or inadequate in terms of energy intake. We might even sit down and eat a normal meal with them to model normal eating.

So Intuitive Eating is best seen as the model of eating that will ultimately become one's own. This happens after there has been a period of time for healing the body physically and shifting the cognitive distortions that rule the mind of someone who has developed an eating disorder as a coping mechanism. We must also strongly say that someone who is seeking help for an eating disorder must also be dealing with the emotional issues that may have been a precursor to the development of this disorder as well as a factor in its maintenance. The appropriate source for this part of the treatment is a psychotherapist who has been trained in eating disorders. A medical doctor who can monitor the physiological state of a patient is also critical in many cases, and, for some, a psychiatrist may be involved to evaluate medication needs.

In our work, we, as nutritionists, are a part of a well-oiled and communicative treatment team. Once the person with anorexia has gained sufficient weight to be able to think clearly and to perceive some of the normal signals of hunger and fullness, or the person with a binge disorder has practiced eating for the body's needs and not primarily for emotional reasons, he or she is able to embark on the path of becoming an Intuitive Eater. Now let's get into the lives of Skylar, Lila, Laurel, Samantha, and a few other of our patients to see how their experiences with dieting led them down the path to their eating disorders. We'll then see how making Intuitive Eating their own has freed them completely from their fear of eating and their fear of unnatural weight gain and, ultimately, has led them to a happier and fuller life experience.

Skylar Skylar was referred for treatment of her "Anorexia" by her psychotherapist at the age of fifty-seven. To look at Skylar at that time, one would see a striking, well-dressed woman who did not look emaciated. Even though she looked somewhat listless and had no sparkle in her eyes, she certainly did not give the image of someone with anorexia nervosa. Yet, the thoughts and behaviors of this woman mimicked those that had imprisoned her from the age of fifteen and had followed her through a hospitalization for anorexia at a weight of 96 pounds, through gradual weight gain over the years, to a weight of 135 pounds.

This weight was achieved with very little increase in caloric intake; instead her metabolism had slowed down over the forty-plus years of her eating disorder, as a result of inadequate calorie input to compensate for her caloric output. Her body sensed a state of starvation and responded by slowing everything down, especially her ability to burn calories. At 5'3" she certainly did not meet the weight-loss criterion of anorexia nervosa, but her pattern of restriction, with its lack of sufficient energy intake, and her obsessive thinking and fear of food and eating, certainly qualified her as having an eating disorder. Skylar's story begins, as it does for so many of our patients who develop anorexia nervosa, with a history of being overweight as a child

The ultimate Ppath toward healing from eating disorders and then being delivered into the world of dieting as a way to "Rescue" her from the fate of obesity. She reported being aware of a sense of being overweight at age ten. At twelve to thirteen she was counting calories with her mother. (As an aside, many well-intentioned, but uninformed parents believe that restricting calorie intake or certain types of food will help their children lose weight and feel better about themselves.

Unfortunately, in most cases, just the opposite occurs. Children end up feeling different, deprived, and frequently rebellious. And, as a result of these feelings, they are ultimately led right into the trap of an eating disorder.) At about the same age that Skylar began counting calories, her family went on a summer visit to her grandfather's home. Two other families with whom her family was very close joined them on this vacation. Within this group were three very thin girls of Skylar's age. Of course, the comparisons began, not only in Skylar's mind, but also by her mother, who was very focused on weight and who told Skylar that she was eating too much. When the family got home at the end of this trip, Skylar was taken to the doctor, who then put her on a regimented diet to lose weight. In subsequent years, Skylar's food intake was carefully watched, except when she went to summer camp. At camp, she would eat freely, but would naturally lose weight from all of the activity. She never felt overweight, as there was no emphasis placed on weight. The summer she turned fifteen; she became excited to go back to camp. It had been a very tough year in school; she knew she would lose weight at camp, and that gave her something for which to look forward.

After the summer, with its accompanying weight loss, Skylar decided to take an active part in continuing her weight loss. She ate no breakfast or lunch, would only eat Jell-O during the day, and at dinner said that she was on a diet. In her home, dieting was praised, so there was no objection to her small food intake with the food she actually ate came anguish and fear. Her solution to these feelings was found in spitting as much of her food as she could into her napkin when no one was watching and then flushing it down the toilet. Skylar's fear and obsessional thinking became so intense that she began to use no water when brushing her teeth, as she was sure that anything that went into her mouth, even water, would make her fat. She never used salt, as she was afraid that that would get into her body and cause her to retain water and become fat. Ultimately, all that she would allow in her body was one apple a day.

She went from 145 pounds to 96 pounds. Now, of course, her mother was angry with her and would try to get her to eat, but she would refuse. Finally, while visiting a friend who was in the hospital, Skylar passed out from malnutrition. She was admitted to the hospital for three to four days and was then discharged to the care of "Dr. Smith," who weighed her, told her she looked like a concentration camp victim and that she would never have children. Little by little, Skylar began to eat moderately. She gradually put on weight until she reached 105 pounds, but was getting on the scale two to three times a day.

Ultimately, she stopped weighing herself and began bingeing on ice cream, which was the main food that she ate. In her twenties, Skylar began using diet pills and diuretics in her frantic attempt to control her weight. When she was thirty-two, Skylar moved to

California, at a weight of 110 to 115 pounds. When she subsequently reached 135 pounds, the powerful force of her anorexia grabbed her again, and she again stopped eating. In her late thirties and early forties, at a weight of 112 pounds, she began to eat again, subsisting mainly on frozen yogurt. Finally, in this state of restriction, having gained almost twenty pounds without increasing her caloric intake or variety of food, living with enormous fear of food and of further weight gain, she began her nutrition therapy. Skylar is now fifty-nine and has spent two years healing her anorexic experience, searching for and finding the Intuitive Eating signals with which she was born, and practicing her new relationship with food.

Today, she eats three meals and two snacks a day. She eats in restaurants regularly, something that previously gripped her with terror, and eats a wide variety of foods. She restricts nothing and actually prefers to eat a normal meal rather than her two pints of frozen yogurt. She exercises consistently, but not excessively and takes in enough calories to sustain her during exercise. This has helped her to build healthy muscle tissue instead of breaking it down due to lack of calories. This has resulted in a faster metabolism as opposed to the slow metabolism that she experienced when she was restricting. Oh, and by the way, Skylar's weight

The Ultimate Path Toward Healing from Eating Disorders 219 now falls in a normal weight range of 120 to 125, which is just right for her 5'3", athletic body—less weight than she was when she was restricting her calories and was afraid to eat! (It is important at this point to restate that weighing oneself is contraindicated in the Intuitive Eating process. Weights are used for medical necessity, especially in the case of anorexia nervosa to assure that patients are not undernourished. Patients are usually weighed backwards in either the physician's office or the nutritionist's office, so that they are not focussed on the numbers. At some point, however, the weight issue often needs to be addressed in a safe environment, to help determine what is healthy and to help the patient come to terms with body acceptance.)

Lila Anorexia is only one serious outcome that can emerge from the world of dieting. Bulimia nervosa, or the pursuit of the elimination of calories after they have been consumed, often becomes the desperate solution to failed dieting. As you have seen throughout the book, there is an inevitable rebound that occurs after someone has restricted—either a particular food, or quantity of food. In fact, nearly half of those with anorexia will develop bulimia, with binge-eating behavior. The rebound can either be physiological, as a result of the secretion of brain chemicals, such as neuropeptide Y and others, or it can be psychological, due to the rebellion that results from deprivation.

More often, we see both physiological and psychological rebound. Once overeating takes hold, subsequent to dieting, patients feel out-of-control and terrified that all of the weight that was lost will return, or, even worse, that they'll end up at a higher weight than before. In this desperation, they will look for ways to rid themselves of the calories consumed from overeating or from a binge. Compensatory mechanisms include excessive, compulsive exercise; vomiting; the use of laxatives, diuretics, or diet pills; or starving for a period of time after overeating. (As a note, laxatives and diuretics mainly remove water from the body, not calories. The resultant dehydration gives someone with bulimia a false sense that she/he has lost weight.

There are serious medical consequences accompanying the overuse of these drugs, as there are with diet pills, purging, and even compulsive exercise.) For Lila, dieting began when she was a senior in high school, as she and her girlfriends were preparing for the prom. Prior to this time, Lila always felt that she was a "Bigger" girl, with bigger legs than her friends had, but she wasn't overly concerned about this. Lila describes this time as one in which she was enjoying the "Bonding" experience of going on a diet together with her girlfriends, so that they would "Look Good" for the prom. The daily meal plan for the girls included an apple for breakfast, salad with vinegar for lunch, and chicken and vegetables for dinner.

They decided that they would do this for one week before the prom to "See what would happen." Lila remembers her weight dropping from 141 pounds on her 5'8" body to 136 pounds in the week—for which she was elated. After the prom came graduation, with a subsequent trip to the Caribbean for three and a half weeks. For the first time in her life, she felt completely free and independent. It was a time for partying, eating, and losing her virginity. She drank many pina coladas and ate lots of French bread and desserts. When she got home, she saw that she had gained back the five pounds plus three to five more. During the summer before college, she continued her overeating, as she was rebounding from her diet experience, at the same time as she was navigating so many emotions: anxiety about her newly found independence and sexuality and her impending move away from home.

At this point Lila had gained a total of fifteen pounds, bringing her to 151 pounds. Immediately after arriving at college, Lila became involved in a relationship with a boy that was to last throughout her college year. She found herself going from a very active, athletic high school student who wasn't worried about life, to an inactive, overindulgent college freshman. She continued overeating, began actual bingeing, and had episodes of secret eating. She found herself thinking, "I can't believe I've eaten so much!" and began purging her food as a way to undo her out-of-control behavior. Since Lila lost no weight as a result of her bulimia, she

never thought of it as a weight control mechanism—it was purely a means of erasing the results of her bingeing. (Note: quite a significant amount of calories are still absorbed, even if you vomit after a binge.) Frequently, the experience of feeling out-of-control and consuming, sometimes, up to five thousand extra calories, can be so horrifying to a person that the impulse to eradicate any remnant of the behavior can become as compulsive as the behavior itself. As one makes purging a regular part of life, the sense of responsibility for one's actions disappears. As we have seen, coping with feelings without using food can be a very difficult challenge for many people.

Bulimia, once discovered, sometimes begins as an exciting alternative to either dealing with feelings or overeating. Patients report feeling as if they're "Getting away with murder." Of course, as bulimia progresses, with its physical and mental side effects and its influence on one's normal pattern of eating, this "Solution" ultimately becomes one's nemesis. Very quickly shame emerges, as hiding the food wrappers, isolating in order to find time for the bingeing, or stealing away to the bathroom when eating in public becomes a daily ritual. By Thanksgiving, Lila's bingeing and purging led her to an all-time high weight of 159 pounds. Although still involved with her boyfriend, she felt insecure about herself and about her weight. She began a hard workout program, alternating periods of starving with binge/purge incidents, which occurred once or twice a week. By the end of freshman year, Lila had lost six pounds, as a result of including exercise in her life, but soon found that she was overexercising.

Before going back to school, she sought the help of a nutritionist, who helped her to curb her bulimia. During sophomore year, she joined a sorority and began a crusade to save her sorority sisters from the dangers of developing an eating disorder. For the rest of her time in college, Lila was able to manage her eating and her exercise, was free of bulimia and maintained a weight of 140 pounds. Unfortunately, after graduation, she moved into an apartment with two roommates, one of whom was an overeater and the other a restrictor. It was a highly emotional year, as she broke up with her college boyfriend and was facing the stress of post-graduate life. As a result, she felt depressed and went back to some of her old behaviors of restricting, then bingeing and purging.

The Ultimate Path Toward Healing from Eating Disorders 223 powerful precursor to bulimia. For Samantha, who was a part of a family overly focused on weight and nutrition, a comment about her weight by her grandfather when she was fifteen sent her off on a roller-coaster ride with bulimia, anorexia, and, ultimately, drug abuse. At 4'11" and 97 pounds, Samantha was a petite, but healthy teenager. On a vacation back east one summer, she gained five pounds, which set off negative comments by her grandfather when he saw her in a bathing suit.

As a result, Samantha perceived herself as terribly overweight, this distorted view of her body has stayed with her since, even though she has never been more than 102 pounds. Fathers and, in this case, grandfathers can affect a young girl's sense of self-esteem often even more than mothers or friends. For girls, male family members can represent the population of men at large. How a father, grandfather, older brother, or close uncle reacts to a young girl's physical appearance can set the stage for a fear that no man will ever find her attractive or that her body is never "Good Enough."

In many instances of eating disorders, sexual abuse can trigger a lifelong sense of shame of one's body and a desire to either starve it to such a small size that it won't be noticed or add layers of fat, so that it will not be seen as attractive. The distortion of the normal body size then becomes an armor or a protection against intimacy and sexuality. There may be a disconnection from the body, so that it no longer is seen as a part of oneself, but rather as an object to manipulate.

For Samantha, there was some subsequent inappropriate sexual attention from this same grandfather, as well as negative body comments— all coming at a very vulnerable time of her life from this powerful male figure. At this time, as Samantha puts it, she had just come from being a "Big fish in a small sea" in her junior high school. Starting a large high school, she felt that she had to prove herself worthy, which frightened her and made her feel out of control. And, like others we've seen, she began to control her food as a way to have something in her life that felt within her power to control. By age nineteen, her dieting behavior led her to bulimia, as it did with Lila. Lila's bulimic episodes were fairly infrequent, as compared to Samantha's experience. Samantha saw bulimia as the answer to all of her problems. Over the years, Samantha was rushed to emergency rooms many times with low potassium levels.

Purging dehydrates the body, and with the purged food and water, comes an imbalance of electrolytes, or chemicals, that help regulate the heart's functioning. Samantha's weight dropped to 68 pounds as a result of her starving and purging behavior, and she was hospitalized in an in-patient setting for the first time. This first hospitalization was just the first of at least a dozen. At age twenty or twenty-one, Samantha started to use cocaine to take away her obsession with food.

She had never been a drinker or a drug user, but she found that cocaine took away her appetite and increased her energy. She continued her cocaine use, off and on, for many years thereafter. Between the ages of twenty-one and twenty-seven, there was never a day in Samantha's life where she was not either behaviorally or mentally obsessed with food. When Samantha began her Intuitive Eating work at twenty-seven, for the first time, she felt a hope that she could be free of bulimia and its accompanying compulsion to abuse food and her body.

At that time, Samantha was bingeing and purging from fifteen to twenty times a day. She was able to reduce her episodes to once a day or once every other day. She learned that she could eat normally and maintain a close to healthy weight in the low 90's, with a plentiful amount of food and normal exercise. Samantha is still a "Work in progress." She has left treatment from time to time before her healing has become complete.

Her drug addiction has reared its ugly head periodically, which has sent her down the road to weight loss and a struggle to regain it. She has had many physical problems, including a heart attack, from which she recovered, and disabling osteoporosis, with constant foot pain, but to Samantha's credit, she has never gone back to the number of bulimic episodes that she had in the beginning of treatment. She is valiantly working in psychotherapy to resolve her lifetime of emotional issues, and she is committed to the philosophy of Intuitive Eating as the model she hopes to fully embrace, as she gets stronger. An eating disorder, when treated with both psychotherapy and nutrition therapy in the early days of its inception, can potentially have a short course, which is resolved without permanent physical and/or psycholog-

The ultimate path toward healing from eating disorders ical damage, unfortunately, for those who go without treatment from professionals experienced in working with eating disorders and Intuitive Eating, or for those who drop out of treatment before they are fully able to embrace the Intuitive Eating philosophy, there can be lifelong suffering and anguish, and even death. On the other hand, let's look at a few cases of patients who were able to catch the eating disorder in its early stages with appropriate treatment and come away more rapidly healed.

Melissa Melissa is a fifteen-year-old high school student who wants, more than anything, to have a boyfriend. She has friends, is a good student, but can't seem to connect with a boy. Her parents are going through a rough time in their marriage, and Melissa can feel the tension. She is also feeling somewhat estranged from her mother, as a result of her normal adolescent attempt to separate and individuate from the parent of her same sex in order to establish an identity of her own. As a child, Melissa always loved food, setting no limits on the amount that she ate. She was young and active and never felt overweight.

In third or fourth grade, she began to notice that some of the girls were thinner than she was and were wearing "Cute clothes that showed off their tummies." At the same time, Melissa started to notice her chubby face and stomach and felt that she didn't fit in. This didn't stop her from overeating, however, as she believed that it was impossible for her to diet. Directly before her graduation from elementary school, Melissa decided she was ready to try to lose some weight, so that she could fit into a special dress for the ceremony.

At this she succeeded and having tasted her first "Success" at weight loss, Melissa looked toward beginning high school. She felt that her extra weight was taking away from her prettiness and decided that she wanted to try to be noticed in order to make an impression; her greatest hope was that she would even find a boyfriend, so began her descent into dieting and then further restriction. As a result of her loneliness and isolation, believing that a boyfriend would fix all of her problems, Melissa was vulnerable to developing anorexia. Since there was no boy who would or could quickly arrive to fix the problems, she plunged furiously into a pursuit to fix and control her body. At fourteen years, Melissa was 5'1" and weighed somewhere between 122 and 125 pounds, a weight that was higher than was expected for her height and body frame and that was achieved by overeating to comfort her feelings.

Four months later, when Melissa began her treatment of both psychotherapy and nutrition therapy, she had dropped to 95 pounds and had lost her menstrual cycle. At that time, she was skipping meals, had obsessional thinking about food and her body, and was engaged in strange exercise behaviors, such as running around her house all day. Through a process of first feeding her starving body, so that her normal signals of hunger and fullness could again emerge and then helping her to challenge her food fears, Melissa was able to gain back enough weight to regain the menstrual cycle which had disappeared for four months. This initial recovery was fairly rapid, taking only about two months of treatment.

Making peace with food was the next critical step in her treatment. She found that when she still held a negative judgment about a particular food or would restrict it, she would overeat when that food was reintroduced. Once a food became demystified, her overeating experiences diminished. Now, a year later, Melissa is maintaining a healthy weight, a normal menstrual cycle, and a comfortable relationship with food. She has learned that her emotions were triggers for her overeating and restricting behaviors, something she was never before able to connect. She is now willing to wait for her feelings to subside when they seem unbearable and knows that what's most important is to take care of herself in healthy and nurturing ways.

Dana Dana's story has some similarities to that of Melissa. A normal eater until she was thirteen, with a normal amount of prepubertal fat, Dana began to feel somewhat self-conscious about her body at about age twelve. Like Melissa, Dana began to compare herself to her classmates, which led her to assess herself as bigger than others were. In the beginning of ninth grade, or her first year of high school, she decided that she

The Ultimate Path Toward Healing from Eating Disorders had to "Do something to make a difference." This thinking, along with the emotions that had arisen accompanying her parents' divorce, a subsequent remarriage by her mother, as well as a heart attack suffered by her mother (from which she recovered) set the stage for eating and body image problems. To complicate matters further, when Dana was at her dad's house, he regularly made comments about portion sizes and often told her that she had "Had Enough" even though she often still felt hungry.

Dana's mom had a natural interest in nutrition and regularly bought low-fat foods. This interest, combined with her dad's investment in the amount of food she ate, promoted for Dana an excessive consciousness about food. Dana began her pursuit of "Making a difference" by cutting out the ice-blended chocolate drinks to which she had regularly treated herself at the local coffee bar. Cutting out one small item after another, she found that she had lost five pounds in three months. Concerned about her behavior, Dana's mother took her to see a nutritionist, who, unfortunately, turned out to be unqualified. Concluding that Dana carried a little extra "Fluff" around her middle, the nutritionist inappropriately and incorrectly told her that her body couldn't handle carbohydrates.

She told her to cut down on her starch intake, to which Dana agreed and then complied further by believing that she should also restrict fruits, and even some vegetables, such as carrots! (Note: In many states, anyone can call him or herself a "Nutritionist," as it has no legal meaning. Be sure that your nutritionist is at minimum a registered dietitian [R.D.]. Dietitians must have at least a bachelor's degree, postgraduate training, pass a national exam, and maintain continuing education.) As anyone reading this can now predict, Dana continued restricting what she ate and how much she ate and began to feel fearful of many foods. Being fueled by her sense of accomplishment, a search for identity, and a sense of control, she continued to restrict. She went on to cut out lunches at school, allowed herself to have only one half a bagel at breakfast, and barely ate anything at dinner. When Dana had at first felt larger than her friends and was observed by the nutritionist to have "Fluff" around her middle; she was all of 113 pounds at 5'4"! Not too many months later, she weighed 93 pounds—a loss of 20 pounds. By the time she reached nutrition therapy in our offices, she was 88 pounds.

Unfortunately, she was so weak, and her thinking was so blurred by malnutrition, it was decided that she needed to be admitted to an intensive day treatment program for eating disorders. (As a note, a journey into the Intuitive Eating process must begins, not just with an openness to its potential for healing, but with a mind that is clear enough to understand what is taught and retain the information. At this point, Dana was far beyond this ability. By the time the arrangements were made for admittance, Dana was down to 81 pounds. Even this treatment was not enough to help, as she continued to starve herself on weekends, when not at the program. Eventually, she was admitted to inpatient treatment at a hospital that had an adolescent eating disorder program.

After six months, she was able to leave the hospital at 110 pounds. As her nutrition improved, Dana began to grow again, until she reached a height of between 5'6" and 5 7 ". She was also able to gain more weight to 128 pounds and see a return of her menstrual cycle, but as one might suspect, this was not the end of Dana's story. Although Dana's weight was restored to one within a normal range, she still held fear of eating certain foods and of eating early in the day. Because of these fears, she subsequently gained another 12 pounds as a result of undereating during the day, coupled with excessive overeating at night. Gaining a total of about 60 pounds in eight or nine months perpetuated a sense of feeling a lack of control of her body.

At the same time, dealing with all of her previous emotional issues, plus the normal issues of being a sixteen-year-old in high school, led her to continue to distract herself from these feelings by focussing on her battle with food and body. Dana's overeating at night finally scared her so much that she began once again to restrict her total caloric intake. After a subsequent loss of 15 pounds in three weeks, Dana was, fortunately, unable to maintain this serious restrictive behavior. She then returned to her pattern of nighttime overeating, regularly set up by daytime undereating, and ended up maintaining her previous weight of 128 pounds. At this point, extremely frustrated and frightened, Dana was open to returning to nutrition therapy. Unhappy with her excessive hunger during the day and the discomfort that resulted from overeating at night, she was

finally ready to make peace with food and eating. Since she was at a healthy weight, she very quickly began practicing the principles of Intuitive Eating and was overjoyed by the results. She learned that by not eating enough for her body's needs during the day, she had quickly fallen into primal hunger and was inevitably set up to overeat at night. As soon as she committed to eating sufficient amounts during the day, the nighttime overeating diminished.

Added to this, once she embraced the belief that no food was her enemy and allowed herself free access to foods she had been avoiding, she found that those foods took a normal balanced place in her eating life. While working on Intuitive Eating principles, she also continued in her psychotherapy with her psychologist, deepening her ability to cope with her feelings without using food for this purpose. Now, as a high school sophomore, Dana, like Melissa, has become a stable Intuitive Eater.

Dana's path had a far more dangerous and frightening slope to climb than Melissa's did. Her introduction to appropriate nutrition therapy expectedly suffered a quick demise, as she was far too malnourished to proceed. She required restoration of weight in an inpatient hospital setting in order to be ready for this journey. Melissa, luckily, began treatment while her mind was still clear enough to understand the potential damage that she was doing to her body and was open enough to see the benefit of Intuitive Eating as a healthy model of eating for her future. For both of these girls, as for others whom we've seen and those yet to be discussed, including one young man, the willingness to change entrenched habits and let go of old coping mechanisms could only begin with trust.

The office of the nutrition therapist must provide an atmosphere of safety and hope. Trust can only be developed when one believes that everything that he or she shares will be heard, absorbed, and not judged. He or she needs to know that the nutrition therapist understands that any behaviors revealed, no matter how dangerous or even life threatening, were developed as a way to cope with a private world that was very scary or lonely or sad. Letting go of these coping mechanisms requires patience, a leap of faith, and a learning of new ways to think about food, body, and life. All of this is possible—these patients are just a few of the many who have healed their eating disorders with this work.

Laurel In the previous case histories, we've seen many influences triggering the development of an eating disorder. Comments by family members frequently have a powerful effect on a young person's body image. School pressures, transitions into new phases of development and life experience often create anxieties that are calmed or even numbed by the overuse of food or avoided by undereating and obsessional thinking about food and body. In Laurel's case, a combination of illness and personal trauma set off her eating disorder. Laurel was a naturally slim girl and a normal eater until she was almost seventeen years old. Just before her seventeenth birthday, she became very ill with tonsillitis, which decreased her normal appetite.

Losing a few pounds led to positive comments by her friends. Liking this attention, Laurel found herself dieting for the first time in her life. She would tell herself that she didn't need "That cookie" or "That bag of chips." One month later, she got sick again, this time with the flu. Once again, she lost more weight and was given even more attention. Soon after this, Laurel discovered that her boyfriend was cheating on her with her best friend—news that understandably devastated her. Feeling betrayed, she completely stopped eating and began to isolate from her friends. In the first week, she felt no hunger and lost even more weight.

After that, hunger returned, but feeling so unhappy, she chose not to eat and began using laxatives in an attempt to feel some semblance of control in her, now, out-of-control life. Deeply concerned about her well-being, her parents sent her to treatment with a psychotherapist with whom she has a wonderful relationship. She was also sent to a nutritionist, with whom she unfortunately did not connect.

She was given a high-calorie meal plan by the nutritionist, was told to weigh and measure her food, and to keep a food log.

Unfortunately, the rapid weight gain with its accompanying refeeding edema (water retention that occurs when eating begins again after a period of starvation) caused so much discomfort and feelings of being out of control with her body that Laurel began purging to get some relief. Ultimately, she stopped all of this, including seeing the nutritionist and any kind of healthy eating. Instead, all she ate was candy!

The Ultimate Path Toward Healing from Eating Disorders 231 At this point, Laurel was referred to nutrition therapy by her psychotherapist. As in other cases previously mentioned, the safety that Laurel felt in this new experience led to a feeling of trust and a willingness to absorb information that would help her to change her thinking about eating and begin the journey to rebuild a healthy relationship with food. Laurel was treated as part of the team in her recovery. She was told that, ultimately, her body was hers to protect and that a decision to get healthy again had to come from within. Clearly, it hadn't worked for her to follow an authoritarian recommendation.

In her new treatment, she felt respected as an individual who was intelligent and capable of making healthy decisions. She also appreciated hearing that everything she had attempted in her eating disorder was done as a coping mechanism, and she began to examine the trade-offs between what she was getting by maintaining her disordered eating and what she was giving up.

She was taught about starvation's effect on her metabolism,

energy levels, immune system, and sleep patterns. She was taught that eating in a balanced way that would be respectful to her body would prevent large blood sugar fluctuations and provide her the nutritional building blocks to make the materials for the building and making of hormones, strong bones, immunoglobulins, muscle tissue, neurotransmitters, and more. Soon, Laurel was able to see that the isolation she was experiencing as a result of her fear of eating in public, along with the potential dangers to her body by maintaining her current patterns was far more frightening than actually learning to eat again.

This time around, however, she began by taking tiny baby steps rather than giant leaps. Adding a bit of protein to her day, such as a string cheese in the morning or some cottage cheese or yogurt at lunch was acceptable to her. It was not too much food to encourage excessive bloating, but it was a step in a healthy direction. Little by little, she added new foods, always working toward a balance of protein, carbohydrates, and fats. She began to include fruits and vegetables, waffles and brown rice and pizza, nuts and beans, beef jerky and avocado. She learned that she could include some "Play Food" in the day without tipping the balance. Little by little, she began gaining weight, with very little physical discomfort. She practiced and rehearsed what it would be like to go to dinner with friends.

Although feeling scared, she took the risk and got through the initial experience, feeling triumphant. Her friendships were renewed, and she accomplished the task of college applications, the joy of the senior prom, and graduation. Today, Laurel is away in her first year at college, preparing and providing food for herself as well as eating out with friends.

She again experiences normal hunger signals and has regained a healthy amount of weight, getting her period again regularly. Laurel has had a few emotionally uncomfortable experiences, which have led her to an initial loss of appetite and a fleeting thought that controlling her eating might give her a sense of emotional control. On the other hand, she very quickly remembers the conversations she had in the early days of her psychotherapy and nutrition therapy and is able to get right back on track. She stays in touch by telephone weekly and feels that this support is an important part of her transition into independence. All of the stories we've told so far were those of girls and women, but eating disorders are not absent in the world of men. Let's now look at one case history of a young man whose eating disorder was not only triggered by some of the same factors as seen before, but was also influenced by the media.

Trevor Trevor is a thirty-one-year-old man whose weight was normal until the age of twelve. Emotional discomfort triggered as a result of being a member of a dysfunctional family as well as problems in school, led him to overeating. Although teased mercilessly by his sister, who called him disparaging names, he blocked this out and remained in denial of his compulsive-eating problem. By the time he was eighteen, Trevor stepped on the scale and found that he was 205 pounds at a height of 5'8" or 5'9".

At this point, Trevor decided that he was going to do something about his weight. His solution was to begin taking laxatives, which he mistakenly thought would produce true weight loss. He knew that both his sister and her friend were taking laxatives with this purpose in mind. He also knew that his mother was regularly using suppositories. As expected, Trevor lost no weight from this dangerous practice and decided to join a health club to see if that would help. Unfortunately, he was lonely and

depressed and was eating most of the time, again, precluding any weight loss. At that point, he read a story in a magazine that said that a particular celebrity was only consuming orange juice as a weight-control method. Impressionable, Trevor decided to try starving himself in the same way. (As a note, many people, especially those suffering from low self-esteem and eating disorders, often worship celebrities and project into them a great deal of power and wisdom.

They often admire their looks and copy their styles of dress and behaviors—a potentially dangerous act!) At twenty, Trevor moved to California, bringing his starving behavior along with him. He began taking college classes in the mornings and would go to the market afterwards to make a salad with non-fat dressing from the salad bar, his only allotted food choice for the day. As time went on, his routine changed to one of allowing himself only a bag of rice cakes per day. He began taking sedatives so that he could sleep all day and avoid feelings of hunger, but his hunger became so intense that it would wake him. Regardless of what Trevor ate, he continued taking laxatives and began to purge. Soon, friends were telling Trevor that he was looking skinny and pale.

This attention, no matter how negative, pleased him deeply. Eventually, the rice cakes were eliminated, and Trevor was in a complete state of starvation. Finding himself in such primal hunger, Trevor one day consumed an entire bottle of ketchup. At this point, realizing how sick he had become, he entered treatment with a psychotherapist, who referred him for nutrition therapy.

Although emaciated, Trevor still saw himself as the fat boy he had been in high school. He didn't believe that he deserved to eat and felt that food was like poison for him. Developing a healthy therapeutic relationship, Trevor slowly took the steps toward becoming an Intuitive Eater. In fact, he even felt so much trust during the first session that he actually bought and ate a bran muffin directly after the session—the first of many steps on his path.

Ten years later, Trevor is now a normal eater. He has come a long way from believing that the simple suggestion to eat was a ridiculous thought and that starving, laxatives, and purging were the only method of weight control for him. He now knows that eating and throwing up doesn't work for him and that consuming balanced meals, eaten regularly throughout the day, speeds his metabolism and allows him to maintain a normal weight of 160 pounds at 5T0".

DEFINING MOMENTS

It is truly immaterial whether an eating disorder happens to a female or a male or whether it begins as a result of dieting to prepare for a prom or as an answer to avoiding painful feelings. What is most important is that one is able to connect with a psychotherapist and a nutrition therapist who understand the psychology of eating disorders and can offer a safe arena for the exploration of the thoughts and feelings that are connected to the patient's relationship with food. Sometimes, during the treatment, there can be one defining moment that can affect the healing process profoundly.

The following are a few vignettes that illustrate defining moments: Kelly is a college senior whose anorexia and bulimia were so severe that she had at one point reached a low weight of 73 pounds at a height of 5'6" and was purging anything that she ate. When she was first seen for nutrition therapy, she had managed to get her weight up to 87 pounds, under the threat of hospitalization, but was still firmly entrenched in her eating disorder. One day during a nutrition therapy session, when Kelly was most resistant to changing her habits, she was asked a question that became critical to her recovery.

She was asked to explain what her greatest fear was in the realm of her nutrition treatment. It was expected that she would say that she was afraid of getting fat. Surprisingly, her answer was not this common response but, rather, that she was afraid of giving up her bulimia. She was regularly using the act of purging as a way to reduce anxiety. As she had never been overweight prior to her eating disorder, and as none of her family members was overweight, Kelly was able to acknowledge that she didn't believe that her body could become too large. This realization became the defining moment that catapulted her leaps and bounds in her recovery. With an extremely depleted physical state, as a result of her malnutrition, she was well aware that her energy levels were very low, that she was isolating from her friends, and that she was having difficulty focussing in school. She was at imminent risk

of being hospitalized if her poor health continued, which, of course, would make continuing in school impossible. But, for the first time, she realized that she didn't have to be afraid of getting fat! At that moment, Kelly became willing to eat again not because she was being externally forced, but because having had an epiphany about her genetics, she decided that she truly wanted to get well and be able to maintain normalcy in her life. She had now become a teammate in her own recovery! Working on the premise that she was not genetically destined to be overweight, Kelly began to take in more food.

Her weight restoration and return of her menstrual cycle was rapid, with an 18-pound weight gain occurring in a three-month period. Along with this came an ability to feel appropriate hunger and fullness again—sensations she hadn't recognized for a very long time. At this point, the time had come to work on refining

Kelly's sense of satisfaction in eating. Recently, when asked if there was any one thing that particularly helped her during this period, Kelly's face lit up, and she said, "Yes, it was your story about eating a chocolate truffle during the movie Chocolat"—one more defining moment! She loved hearing about the sensual experience of slowly tasting and savoring a delicious piece of chocolate while watching a film about a chocolate shop in France. She had also seen the film, wishing that she could enjoy the chocolate—a food she had forbidden for herself.

With a commitment to make peace with food, as well as trust in her nutrition therapist as a role model, Kelly began an exploration of all the foods, including chocolate, which she had restricted for years! A year and a half later, Kelly has maintained the original weight that she regained and eats with a freedom that she hasn't felt since before her anorexia began.

Her bulimic episodes have drastically decreased, mainly because a large percentage of her bulimic behavior had been triggered by primal hunger and a belief that she was not allowed to eat many of the foods that she loved.

She is continuing to work with her psychiatrist to find ways of coping with her anxiety without using food, with the goal of ultimately letting go of the bulimia completely. Delia, a beautiful and striking six-foot-tall twenty-three-year-old, had been in a battle with food all of her life. Taking after her father's side of the family, which tended toward a stocky build, Delia always felt selfconscious about her body in comparison with her ultra-thin sister and mother. She began dieting at age fourteen, beginning a roller-coaster ride of drastic weight fluctuations, diet pills, food restriction, compulsive overeating, laxative abuse, and purging, which lasted until she began nutrition therapy at the age of twenty-two.

In her first session, when Delia was asked about her favorite foods, she mentioned many healthy foods, such as beans and soups and vegetables and meat, and then, guiltily, acknowledged that she liked candy, but could only eat it in excess. As the Intuitive Eating process was explained to Delia, and she heard that she would always be able to eat any food that she desired, even candy, a sense of disbelief, followed by a sense of calm took her over.

Delia has since said that this moment of hope was one that has changed her life forever. She knew that all of her attempts at weight loss had not worked and decided that if she was going to be "Fat" all of her life, she might as well forget about her body and just "Feel Good." She left the office with a resolve to quit dieting once and for all. Immediately, she experienced a quieting of her mind and a feeling of peace that she had never remembered feeling in relationship to eating.

Although past experiences with losing weight gave her a temporary feeling of well-being, this couldn't compare with what she ultimately has felt as an Intuitive Eater. After a year and a half of this work, Delia still loves candy, but, now, she doesn't need to eat the whole box—in fact, she never even thinks about it. Eating has become a pleasurable experience. As she follows her hunger and fullness and taste preferences, she gets satisfaction from her meals, enjoys the small amount of play food that she desires, and never feels stuffed. All is quiet on the front of Delia's war with food and body, and, by the way, she has begun to lose weight—what a surprise! Kathy fought the same mental battle as Delia, even though she was not overweight when she sought nutrition therapy. An athlete all of her life, Kathy was muscular and toned, weighing, most of her life, 135 pounds at 5'4". At one point in her life, feeling miserable in her job and using food to deal with her stress, she had reached a high weight of 152

Readiness For Intuitive Eating

Eating disorders can take from a few months to many years for healing to take place. This depends on how long you've had the eating disorder, when you're ready to seek help, and other mitigating factors. It's important to be patient with yourself, it's unlikely that anyone with an eating disorder can dive straight into Intuitive Eating. If you start too soon, without professional help, you may end up feeling scared, frustrated, and overwhelmed. Here are some of the indicators of when you are ready to move into work on Intuitive Eating.

Remember, this should be done in conjunction with your health-care team:

- Biological Restoration and Balance. If you have anorexia, this means weight restoration. It's not realistic to expect yourself to be able to hear hunger signals, let alone honor hunger and fullness. If you have bulimia or a binge eating disorder, this means moving from a pattern of chaotic eating to regular meals. Regardless of the eating disorder, it will usually take some sort of eating plan with a nutrition therapist to get you back into balance.

- Recognition That the Eating Disorder Is Not About Weight or Food, but Rather Something Deeper. Once you begin to accept this . . . eating will move into the realm of self-care rather than a staunch attempt at defending its existence.

- Ability to Recognize and Willingness to Deal with Feelings. As you are able to identify and appropriately cope with your feelings, the need to turn to eating disorder behaviors will decrease.

- Ability to Identify Your Wants and Needs. As you are able to identify your wants and needs, the less you will need your eating disorder behaviors to fill that unmet void.

- Ability to Risk. As your body begins to heal both physically and psychologically, you will be ready to take and tolerate risks with your eating. For someone with anorexia, it may simply be eating a food without knowing its exact calorie content. For someone with bulimia, it might be savoring chocolate for the first time.

In the healing of a serious eating disorder, we often see periods of time when the symptoms of the eating disorder return. These times are associated with increased periods of stress, which are greater than the person's ability to cope. When this happens; one needs to see the return of symptoms as a red flag, which is not to be ignored. It represents a need to seek help in order to get back on the path of healing and Lila did just that. She sought a psychologist at an eating-disorder clinic who helped her to stop purging. Directly afterwards, she began doing the work required to help her find her way back into Intuitive Eating.

Although she had had a respite from her eating disorder during her last three years of college, she had not truly made peace with food. She had become a careful eater, and a diligent exerciser. As her stress levels increased dramatically, she again sought the behavior of controlling her food as a way of giving her a false sense of control of her life.

She also began overeating again, as a way of comforting herself and numbing her pain. And, once again, the bulimia had returned. Through following the steps of Intuitive Eating, including a commitment to never diet or restrict again, Lila was able to discover that eating primarily for hunger, and respecting her body's signal of fullness, gave her an inner sense of empowerment. Choosing to eat what was appealing to her allowed her to receive satisfaction from her meals. She began to spend time with her feelings, rather than pushing them down, and found that by developing her "Emotional Muscle," she was far better able to cope with life than she had ever been when maintaining bulimic behavior. Today, Lila is a happily married woman with a thriving career. She eats intuitively, includes healthy exercise in her life, and, although she doesn't weigh herself, she wears clothes that fit her better than they did in high school.

CONCLUSION

HONOR YOUR HEALTH—GENTLE NUTRITION

Make food choices that honor your health and taste buds while making you feel well. Remember that you don't have to eat a perfect diet to be healthy. You will not suddenly get a nutrient deficiency or gain weight from one snack, one meal, or one day of eating.

1. It's what you eat consistently over time that matters; progress, not perfection, is what counts.

2. Consider the tenets of food wisdom: variety, moderation, and balance. As with exercise, consider nutrition as your passport into feeling good.

3. Feed your metabolism. Be sure to stoke your metabolic fire by getting sufficient fuel throughout the day by eating whenever you're hungry.

4. Eat plenty of whole grains, fruits and vegetables, and beans for their fiber content, so your digestive tract works well. They're also a powerhouse of vitamins, minerals, and phytochemicals.

5. Eat sufficient protein, but not too much, for cellular repair and production of hormones, enzymes, hair, nails, etc.

6   Eat plenty of carbohydrates and sufficient calories so your protein can be used as a protein source and not be burned as an energy source.

7   Take in an adequate amount of dairy products to get enough calcium to keep your bones strong. Drink plenty of water to aid digestion, prevent constipation, have sufficient blood volume, and cleanse your kidneys.

MODELING HEALTHY ATTITUDES FOR YOUNG PEOPLE

Set a positive example of a healthy and balanced relationship with food. Don't talk about or behave as if you are constantly dieting; encourage eating a broad variety of foods in response to body hunger. Don't equate food with positive or negative behavior. The dieting parent who says she was "Good" today because she didn't Eat Much" teaches that eating is bad, and that avoiding food is good. Similarly, "Don't eat that it will make you fat" teaches that being fat makes one unlikable. Learn about and discuss with your sons and daughters the dangers of trying to alter their body shape through dieting. Trust your children's appetites; never try to limit their caloric intake unless requested to do so by a physician for a medical problem.

Help children accept and enjoy their bodies and encourage physical activity. Love, accept, acknowledge, appreciate, and value your children out loud no matter what they weigh. Convey to children that weight and appearance are not the most critical aspects of their identity and self-worth. Do not communicate the message that you cannot dance, swim, wear shorts, or enjoy a summer picnic because you do not look a certain way or weigh a certain amount.

Notice often and in a complimentary way how varied people are—how they come in all colors, shapes, and sizes. Show appreciation for diversity and a respect for nature. Link respect for diversity in weight and shape with respect for diversity in race, gender, ethnicity, intelligence, etc. Educate your children about the existence, the experience, and the ugliness of prejudice and oppression—whether it is directed against people of color or people who are overweight.

Devote yourself to raising non-sex-stereotyped children by modeling and living gender equality. Develop a historical perspective on the politics of the control of women's bodies. Work toward and speak out for human rights: to fair pay, to safety, to respect, and to control of their bodies. Demonstrate a respect for people as they age, in order to work against the cultural glorification of youth and a tightly controlled ideal body type. Take people seriously for what they say, feel, and do, and focus less on the way they look.

Give children the same opportunities and encouragement (in assignment of chores, choosing a sport, etc.) and avoid restricting children to gender-specific activities. Remain close to and supportive of your children as they experiment and struggle with body image, grooming and cosmetic issues, flirtatiousness and sexuality, etc. Talk to your children about the way body shape and sexuality are manipulated by the media and struggles to conform or not to conform.

Build self-esteem. The most important gift adults can give children is self-esteem. When adults show children that they value and love them unconditionally, children can withstand the perils of childhood and adolescence with fewer scars and traumas. Self-esteem is a universal vaccine that can immunize a youngster from eating problems, body image distortion, exercise abuse, and many other problems. Providing self-esteem is the responsibility of both parents.

Encourage children to talk openly and honestly and really listen to them. Encourage open communication and teach children how to communicate. Recognize that sociocultural pressures surrounding drugs, sexuality, body image, and perfectionism require great character strength, self-assurance, and decision-making in young children. Let them know that their opinions and feelings are valued. Encouraging young people to assert themselves helps them say no to pressures to conform. Feeling loved and confident allows them to accept that they are unique individuals.

Encourage critical thinking. The only sure antidote to the tendency to conform to the powerful seduction of the media and peer pressure is the ability to think critically. Become a critical consumer of the media—pay attention to and openly challenge media messages. Talk with your children about the pressures they see, hear, and feel to diet and to "Look Good." Parents have to encourage critical thinking early, and educators have to continue the mission. We need to teach kids how to think, not what to think, and to encourage them to disagree, challenge, brainstorm alternatives, etc.

Develop a value system based on internal values. Help children understand the importance of equating personal worth with care and concern for others, wisdom, loyalty, fairness, self-care and self-respect, personal fulfillment, curiosity, self-awareness, the capacity for relationships, connectedness and intimacy, individuality, confidence, assertiveness, a sense of humor, ambition, motivation, etc. Model this value system; examine, explore, and, if necessary, modify any appearance expectations you have about your child or the children you work with (e.g., 'will they grow up to be pretty?').

Teach children about good relationships and how to deal with difficulties when they arise. People sometimes use food to express or numb themselves instead of dealing with difficult feelings or relationships. Because of messages that suggest that the perfect body will dissolve all relationship problems, young people often put energy into changing their bodies instead of their feelings or their relationships.

Be aware of some of the warning signs of eating disorders. Understand that these warning signs can appear before puberty. Watch for: refusing typical family meals, skipping meals, comments about self and others like "I'm too fat; they're too fat," clothes shopping that becomes stressful, withdrawal from friends, irritability and depression, or any signs of extreme dieting, bingeing or purging.